Antonio dos Santos Rodriguez

Phytotherapy, with Brazilian Herbal Medicines

Antonio dos Santos Rodriguez

Phytotherapy, with Brazilian Herbal Medicines

A Study of the Proof and Effectiveness of Brazilian Herbal Medicines, for Therapy or the Classroom

ScienciaScripts

Imprint

Cover image: www.ingimage.com

This book is a translation from the original published under ISBN 978-613-0-16135-4.

Publisher:
Sciencia Scripts
is a trademark of
Dodo Books Indian Ocean Ltd. and OmniScriptum S.R.L publishing group

120 High Road, East Finchley, London, N2 9ED, United Kingdom
Str. Armeneasca 28/1, office 1, Chisinau MD-2012, Republic of Moldova, Europe
Printed at: see last page
ISBN: 978-620-8-28670-5

SUMMARY

To my patients and students, for them and by them.

To all the professionals who helped me so much in carrying out this work.

To my wife and daughters who have been so tolerant of me.

ACKNOWLEDGMENTS

I thank God first for the opportunity he has given me to serve.

To Prof. Dr. Sumie Hoshino Shimizu, Pharmacist and Professor at the University of Sâo Paulo, the main supporter of this work, for her unconditional support and friendship.

To Prof. Dr. Ieda Maria Magalhâes Laurindo, Collaborating Professor at FMUSP and Assistant Physician at the Rheumatology Outpatient Clinic of the Hospital das Clinicas of the Faculty of Medicine of the University of São Paulo, for all her support in selecting and monitoring the patients.

To Prof. Nidia Denise Pucci, head nutritionist in the Nutrition and Dietetics Division of the Urology, Nephrology and Obstetrics outpatient units of the Central Institute of the Hospital das Clinicas of FMUSP, for all her support during the classes of the Specialization Course in Clinical Nutrition and her suggestions for this work.

To Prof. Maria de Lurdes do Nascimento. PhD and MSc in Public Health from the School of Public Health at USP, Coordinator of the Interdisciplinary Team of the Geriatrics and Gerontology Service at the Hospital do Servidor Pùblico Estadual, Specialist in Clinical Nutrition and Hospital Administration and University Professor, for all her support during the classes of the Specialization Course in Geriatrics and Gerontology and her suggestions for the completion of this work.

To Prof. Celso Ricardo Fernandes de Carvalho, PhD and MSc from the USP School of Medicine, Professor at FMUSP, Physiotherapist at the Pulmonology Outpatient Clinic of the Hospital de Clinicas of the School of Medicine of the University of São Paulo, for all his help with patients at the USP Hospital de Clinicas and support in my Master's degree at FM-USP, as well as tips for this work.

To everyone who, by taking on other tasks that I had to do, allowed me to find the time to devote to this work.

1 BRAZILIAN HERBAL MEDICINES: HOW TO IDENTIFY A PLANT

When we talk about a plant, we usually use its popular name, but the same plant can be known by different names depending on where it is found, for example, Erva de Santa Maria is known in northeastern Brazil as Mastruz. Sometimes different plants are given the same name, which can cause serious confusion, for example Espinheira Santa is also known as Cancerosa and is a plant with low toxicity, however there is another plant also known as Cancerosa or Leiterinha which is toxic and its latex ("milk" that comes out when the branches or leaves are removed) can cause burns when in contact with the skin.

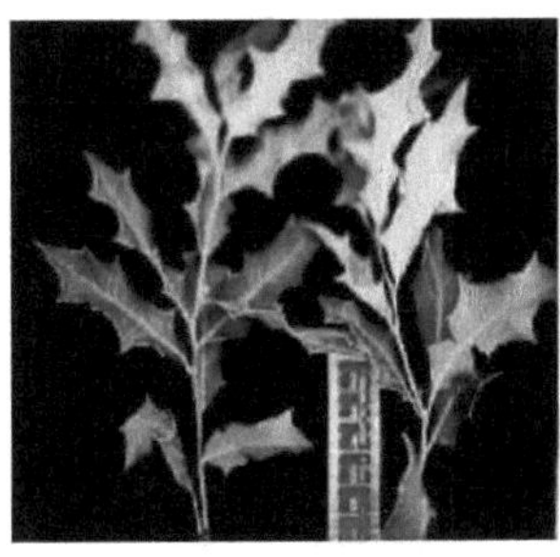

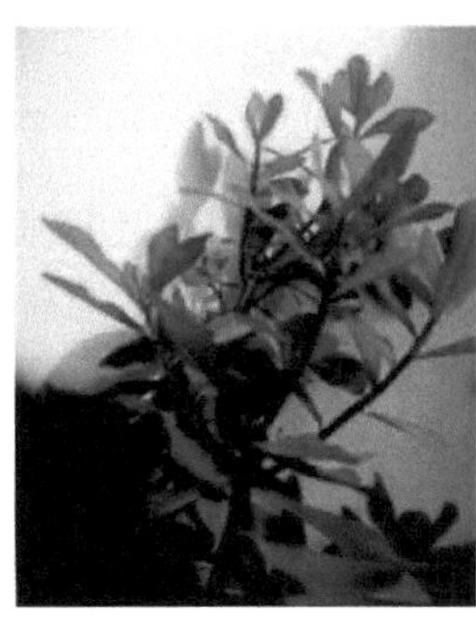

Popular Name: Espinheira Santa **Scientific Name:** Cancerosa or : *Maytenus ilicifolia*

Popular **NameScientific Name**: Cancerosa or Leiterinha: *Philiberthia cuspidata*

Plants can also be known by their scientific name, in which case each plant has a single scientific name, which is written in Latin and consists of two parts: the first is the genus and the second the species, followed by the name of the author of the name, who first identified the plant.

Thus, Espinheira Santa may have more than one popular name, but it only has one scientific name:

Maytenus ilicifolia *Martius*

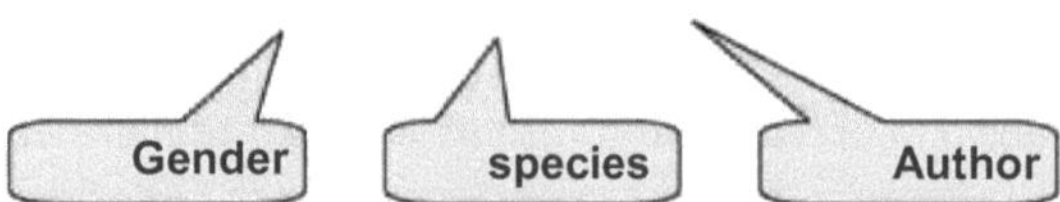

In this course we present technical data sheets for fruits, herbs and spices, in which we see the popular name by which they are best known and the scientific name. When we buy a tea in the supermarket or pharmacy, we will see the popular name and the scientific name on the packaging, so every time we look for information about a plant, we should always look for the scientific name, to avoid confusion. When in doubt, contact the Botany Department of a university. **Attention!**

Do not use a plant as a remedy, especially if you are going to ingest it, without being sure that it is in fact the recommended species.A medicinal plant should only be used when it is well known. Never use unknown plants or those of dubious identity, as serious accidents can occur.

Be sure! Get to know the plants well before you decide to add them to your family pharmacy. Ask, study, question until you're sure!

PART USED AND TIME OF COLLECTION

A plant is a living being and is therefore constantly producing substances which, in the plant, fulfill a function and when used in people can help cure a disease. These substances that have pharmacological activity are called active principles. The active principles responsible for the plant's activity are not always known, although their activity can be scientifically proven.

As a living plant, it is subject to the action of the environment (light, water, temperature, soil and altitude) and can change its composition, either failing to produce certain active ingredients or producing them in greater or lesser quantities.

You need to know in which part of the plant there is the greatest amount of active ingredients and at what time of year this part should be collected. In the technical data sheets for fruit, herbs and spices, we indicate the part to be used. Sometimes the same plant can have different active ingredients, depending on the part used, and therefore has different indications. For example, the peel of the Pomegranate fruit is indicated as having an antiseptic action, while the bark of the stem has an action against the solitary worm (*Tenia solium*).

We collect the part of the plant when its metabolism means that the amount of active ingredients is greatest in that part.

In general, the collection of:

- Leaves: should be before flowering, when the first buds start to appear;

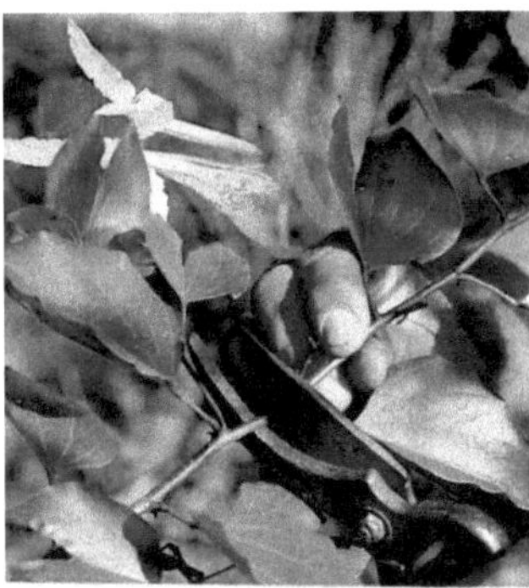

- Flowers: when they open completely, you should observe when the bees are going into the flower, because after pollination the flower *already* starts to "turn" into fruit and the active ingredients can move around;

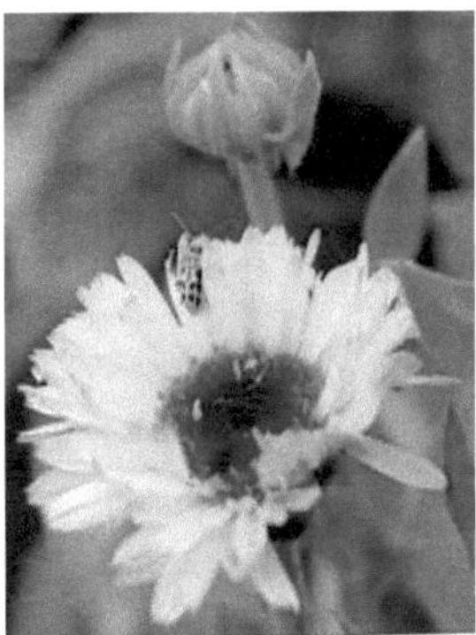

- Roots or rhizomes: at the end of the growing season (fall);

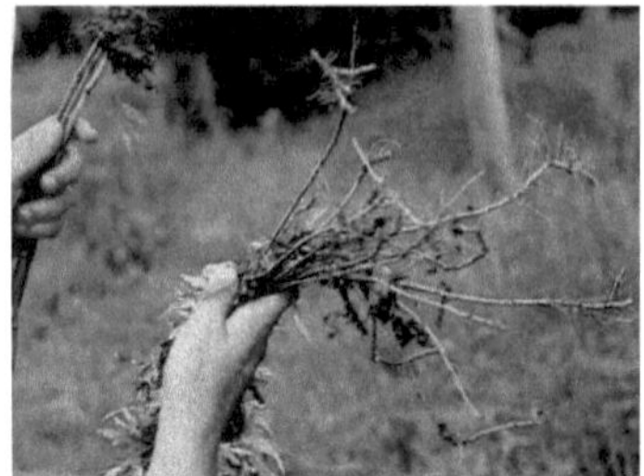

- Fruits: when they are fully developed, at the beginning of ripening;
- Seeds: wait until the end of the plant's cycle, when they are ready to be sown;
- Trunk bark: should be removed in the drier season, as it accumulates a lot of water during the rainy season;
- Aerial parts (above ground): collect the whole plant when it is at the beginning of flowering with the first buds and don't pull out the root;

Attention!

- When collecting leaves, never take more than half of the leaves on the plant. When collecting flowers, fruit and seeds, leave enough to allow the species to multiply. When collecting bark, never collect around the trunk, only on one side;
- We shouldn't collect plants with diseases (spots, fungi, etc.) or insects, as they can be harmful to our health;

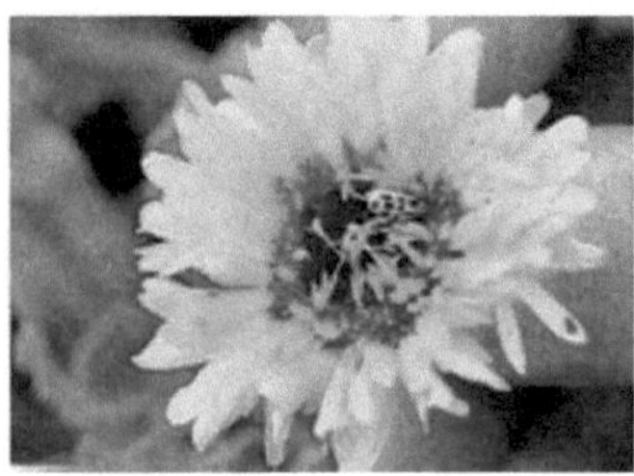

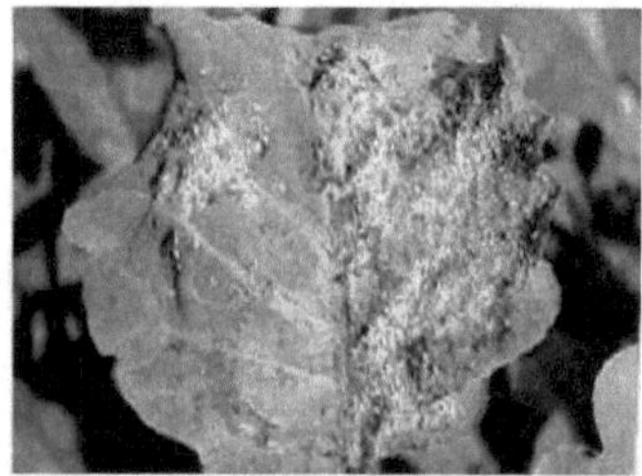

- We must use suitable tools so that we don't harm the plant we've collected or the one that remains alive (as this makes it easier for the cut to heal). We use scissors for leaves, flowers and fruit, a knife for the bark and a shovel for the roots, which should be removed whole when possible.
- When there isn't a lot of plant at the place of collection, we should only collect a quantity that allows the plant to develop and continue multiplying;

- The place where the fruit, herbs and spices are collected should be clean, away from factories, sewers and streets with lots of cars, as the plants could be contaminated. Plants on which pesticides have been applied should also not be eaten.
- We should change the collection site from one year to the next so that the plants have time to recover;
- Harvested material should not be piled up, as this can cause it to become discolored, and it should not be placed directly on the ground;

2 PLANT DATA SHEET

National Bilberry

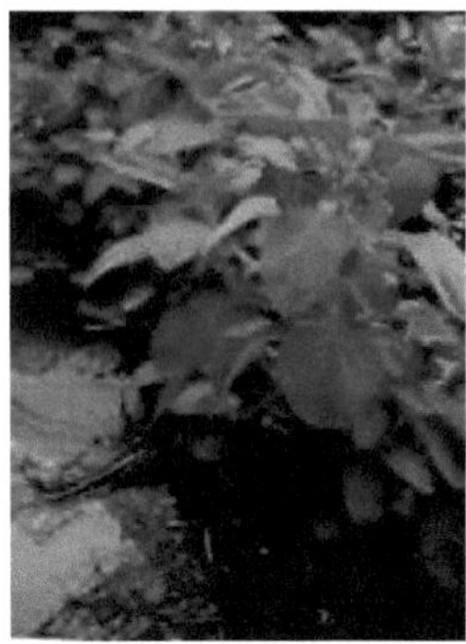

Scientific name:

Plectranthus barbatus Andr.

Popular Names:

Malva Santa, Sete Dores, Boldo, Boldo de jardim; Boldo Silvestre, Malva Amarga, Sete Sangrias, Boldo Brasileiro.

Toxicity:

Large doses or prolonged use cause gastrointestinal irritation and a rise in blood pressure.

Indication	Form of use	Dosage
- Anti-acid, - Anti-ulcer, - Poor digestion; - Heartburn, stomach upset, - Hangover Digestive stimulant	Infusion: 4 to 6g of fresh leaves or 1 to 3g of dried leaves in a cup of boiling water. Maceration. Grind 2 to 3 green leaves (4 to 6g) in 1 cup of water.	Optionally take 2 to 3 cups of tea , sweetened or not.

Chamomile

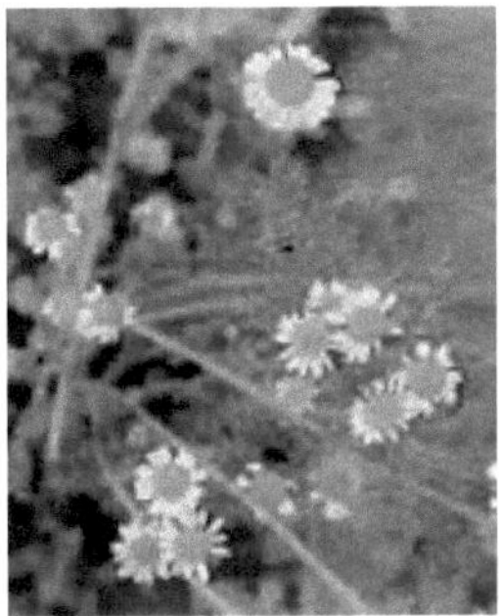

Scientific name:

Matricaria recutita L. Rauschert..,

Popular Names:

Matricaria, manzanilla

Toxicity:

Prolonged and repeated contact with the plant can cause contact dermatitis.

Indication	Form of use	Dosage
- Gingivitis - Canker sores - Sore throat	Mouthwash and gargle: use the infusion Infusion: 2 teaspoons of flowers in 1 cup of boiling water.	3 times a day 1 cup of tea, 3 times a day
- Indigestion - Motion sickness - Intestinal gas - Belly pain	Infusion: as mentioned above	1 cup 3 times a day
- inflamed - Injuries Eczema - Rashes -	Bath: use the infusion after it has cooled down Compress: use the infusion after it has cooled down Ointment Oil	4-5 times a day Apply 4 times a day

Acne burns - Conjunctivitis - -		
- Hemorrhoids	Bath: use the infusion after it has cooled.	4-5 times a day

Coriander

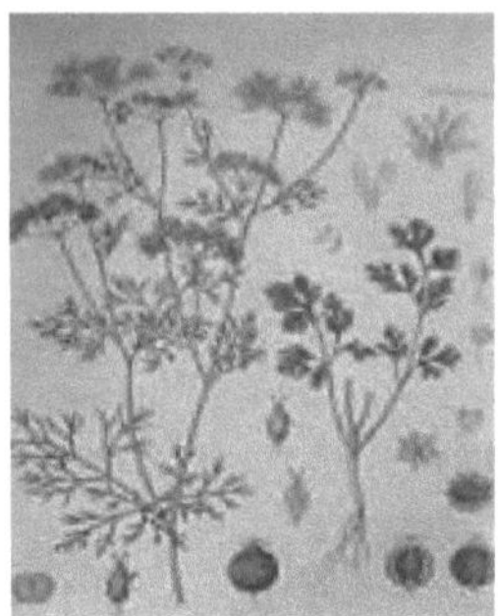

Scientific name:

Coriandrum sativum L.

Toxicity:

Essential oil in high doses can cause convulsions

indication	Form of use	Dosage
Digestive, carminative, stomach pain, intestinal colic and menstrual colic	Salad: used as a dressing 6 g fresh leaves Infusion Tincture: 100 g of fresh leaves in 500 ml of diluted alcohol (2 parts pure alcohol and 3 parts water).	2 x/day 1 cup 3 times a day after meals 1 teaspoon 1 x /day
Joint pain/ Muscle pain	Oil Ointment	Apply locally 3 x/day
Diuretic/ Hypoglycemic	Infusion	1 cup 3x/day

Lemongrass

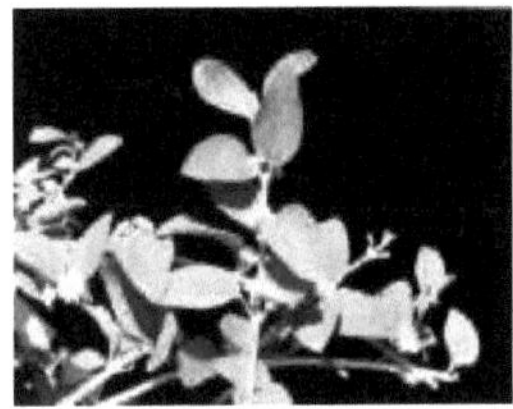

Scientific name:

Lippia alba (Mill.) N. E. Br.

Popular names:

False Melissa, Brazilian Lemon Balm, Fever Tea, Lemon Balm, Lemon Sage, Sàlvia, Flu Sàlvia.

Toxicity:

The literature consulted shows no toxicity to date.

Indication	Form of use	Dosage
Bellyache -	Infusion: 10 leaves (4g) in a cup of water	Take when necessary
- Digestive	Infusion	Take after a meal
Colds, bronchitis,-respiratory infections	Tincture: 100g of leaves to half a liter of diluted alcohol (3 parts alcohol and 2 parts water). Inhalation: use the infusion	Massage onto the chest once a day Inhale once a day
- - Soothing Insomnia	Dye	1 teaspoon 3 times a day
- After childbirth	Infusion	After cooling the tea, make a sitz bath

Sweetgrass

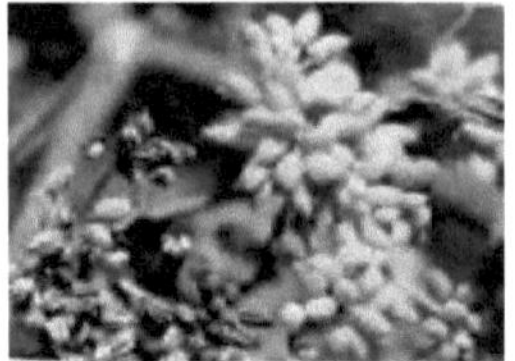

Scientific name:

Pimpinella anisum L.

Popular Name:

Green anise

Toxicity:

The alcoholic extract can be abortifacient, cause alterations and disorders in the fetus, cause irritation and redness on the skin and even convulsions in children, so it should be used with caution.

Indications	Form of use	Dosage
- Digestive - Intestinal gas - Laxative .	Infusion: 1 g of the fruit in 1 cup of boiling water	1 cup after meals.
- Expectorant, cough, asthma and bronchitis Soothing -	Infusion	1 cup, 3 times a day.
- Acne, wounds	- Bath: use the infusion on the affected area	3 times a day

Guava tree

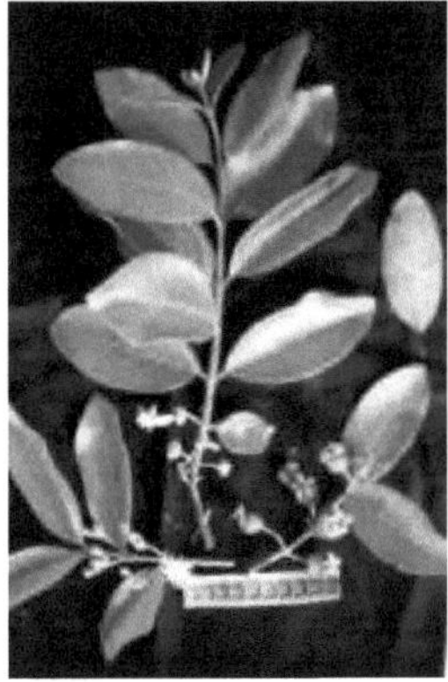

Scientific name:

Psidium guajava L

Popular Name:

Araça-Goiaba, Araça-Guabà, Araçù-Guaçù, AraçùUaçu, Guaiaba-vermelha, Guaiava

Toxicity:

The presence of tannins makes it inadvisable to use this plant internally for a long time, as it can cause disorders due to poor food absorption.

Indication	Form of use	Dosage
Dysentery, diarrhea	Infusion: 30 g of young leaves in 500 ml of water	Take 1 to 2 cups of tea a day.
Mouth sores, gingivitis, sore throat, thrush	Mouthwash and gargle: use the infusion	Rinse or gargle 2 to 3 times a day. Take 2 cups of tea a day.
Skin wounds	Bath: use the infusion on the affected area	Wash the wound 3 times a day.
Vaginal candidiasis, trichomoniasis	Bath	Bathe 3 times a day

3 MEDICINAL PLANTS: HISTORY, TRADITION AND CURRENT EVENTS

Throughout history, man has always sought to overcome his ills. Numerous stages have marked the evolution of the art of healing. However, it is difficult to delimit them exactly, since the art of healing was, for a long time, associated with magical, mystical and ritualistic practices. At all these stages, healing practices used medicinal plants.

Initially, man was concerned with the immediate relief of the symptoms of illness, especially pain, and later he dedicated himself to understanding how the body worked in health and disease. And to cure it, he made use of what nature had to offer, especially the use of plants.

Man has always observed how animals use plants and the effects they can have. If a certain plant had a beneficial effect on the animal, it was deduced that it would certainly have the same effect on man.

But the knowledge of how to use plants as medicines was not only acquired by observing animals. Man has always used plants as a source of food and observed the effects they had on his body. As a result, he began to sort out which plants had nutritional, medicinal and toxic properties, etc.

Later, he began to search for medicinal plants in a systematic way. For a long time, this search was marked by the theory of signatures. It was believed that in nature there were elements capable of curing all ailments and that these elements had a sign, a clue capable of identifying them with their therapeutic function. The main sign would be the similarity of the shape and color of the plant or its parts with the organs affected by the diseases.

This is how the therapeutic potential of medicinal plants was discovered. At first, intuitively, and later through systematic experimentation.

As an example of the intuitive and experimental process used by man in the early days of civilization, we have the fable that says that a shepherd took his goats out to pasture every day. While grazing, he noticed that the animals were eating the fruits of some of the plants that were there and that, after a while, they became completely euphoric and ran around the fields. So he decided to eat these fruits and in doing so he was able to stay awake and say his prayers. Later, the fruits of this plant were roasted into a powder and used to prepare a tea, which became used worldwide. Thus, according to tradition, the use of coffee was discovered.

In ancient times, there was a belief in the magic of the plant kingdom, which could be discovered and used through empirical knowledge of plants. This belief was appropriated by alchemy and occultism, which attributed to plants an astral field capable of interfering with the physical and spiritual body that oscillated from good to evil, from love to hate, from health to illness, from life to death.

This understanding has been passed down from generation to generation and to this day, in some religions, both Eastern and Western, there is a belief in the magical power of plants, to the point where some of them are considered sacred plants, from which preparations are made that are capable of provoking a state of trance that connects their users to spiritual entities. In our culture, we can mention jurema preta and ayuasca.

Whether used for mystical purposes or not, over time plants have gained respectability in all civilizations for demonstrating their therapeutic potential in the health-disease process, as well as their toxic properties.

The first written information on medicinal plants was found in excavations in Mesopotamia in 1872 and dates back to the 16th century B.C. They are the Ebers Papyrus, an Egyptian writing that includes more than 700 prescriptions with natural products, mainly plants, among them garlic, ricin, myrrh, aloe, flax, thyme, cannabis, fennel, saffron, among others.

In fact, plants were the first source of resources for intervening in human illness. The Bible refers to the use of garlic, pennyroyal, cumin, mint, nettles, etc.

The Egyptians made a great contribution to phytotherapy by using plants not only to cure illnesses, but also to embalm bodies and for religious rituals. The onion bulb was considered a symbol of the universe and was consecrated to the goddess Mother Iris. The Egyptians used many herbal preparations with aromatic, antiseptic and cosmetic properties, as well as cultivating purgative, diuretic and vermifuge plants, etc.

The Assyrians cultivated various plants that served as raw materials for the preparation of tinctures, ointments and aromatic waters, while the Hebrews used the plants they cultivated for their ceremonies and offerings, such as myrrh.

In China, there have been reports of healing with plants since 3000 BC. For this reason, China is considered to be the cradle of the use of plants with medicinal properties. The literature mentions that Emperor Shen Nung, considered the Chinese Hippocrates, studied and reported the therapeutic and toxic power of more than 300 species of plants in the Book of Herbs.

In ancient Rome, garlic was used to scare away evil spirits and soldiers in ancient Greece carried garlic in bags in their caps to protect themselves from witchcraft and misfortune.

Hippocrates, considered to be the father of Western medicine, believed that the prevention and cure of diseases were to be found in nature, and that it was only up to man to decode them. With this understanding, he compiled in his work, *Corpus Hippocraticum*, a set of information about the treatment of illnesses with herbal remedies. He was followed by many others, such as Theophrastus, Pliny, Asclepiades, Pelacius, Dioscorides, etc.

Dioscorides (40-90) made the first systematic compilation of plants in his work De Matéria Médica. In it, 579 plants are catalogued and 4,700 uses and forms of action of these plants are described. This book was of great importance to European medicine until the 17th century.

India is the country that, alongside China, has a great tradition in the use of medicinal plants, which form the basis of Ayurvedic medicine. There, several works have been written on herbal medicines such as sandalwood, cinnamon, cardamon and on the preparation of elixirs, tinctures, essences, juices, extracts, etc.

It was in the second century after Christ that plants became more widely used in therapy. This was due to the tireless efforts of several scholars such as Galen, who wrote several works and gained notoriety within pharmacology for the preparation of his formulations, today known as Galenic formulas.

With the fall of the Roman Empire, medical knowledge was discredited because it was no longer able to meet the demand for existing pathologies. During this period, the keeping and reproduction of writings related to medicine was confined to monasteries, which began to act as depositories of medical knowledge. Large medicinal gardens were common in these places.

The church, which already wielded a great deal of power in relation to spiritual matters, came to hold power over the physical body, since it was the religious who were responsible for transcribing the records. The population, however, was totally devoid of care and began to develop healing practices on their own. It was within this context that popular medicine emerged, permeated with magical practices exercised by healers, witches, travelers and the population in general.

In the Middle Ages, there was a re-dimensioning of popular and scholarly knowledge about plants. During this period, the theory of signatures gained prestige. It was believed that the cure was to be found in nature and that it was up to man to decode the signs. For example, plants shaped like beans, which is the shape of the kidneys, were used to treat a disease affecting the kidneys. For diseases of the brain, plants shaped like walnuts, etc.

The 16th century saw major changes and innovations in the arts, philosophy and science, culminating in the Renaissance.

During this period, three factors contributed to the consolidation of ***herbal*** medicine: ***the advance of botany, which was boosted by the study of plant classification; the spread of herbalism, with the creation of herbariums and medicinal plant gardens, mainly at universities; and the discovery and exchange of medicinal plants between different regions, due to the great navigations and the establishment of trade routes.***

In Brazil, the first records of the use of plants date back to the 16th century and correspond to the manuscripts of Fr. Anchieta. In these, he reports that in the fishing trips made by the Indians who lived here, the fish would surface just by touching the water with vines. This was later explained by the discovery of the narcotic and healing substances contained in the plants they used. The Jesuits played a major role in spreading the indigenous knowledge of medicinal plants to the general population.

Throughout the history of the colony, the use of medicinal plants native to Brazil was consolidated with those brought by the Portuguese and Africans, in conjunction with religious practices. The movement of people exploring the interior of the country, in search of gold or Indians for enslavement, was fundamental in the exchange of information about the use of medicinal plants.

It is also worth highlighting some scholars who have compiled the plants used by different communities, in publications that are very important as historical and scientific sources on the use of medicinal plants. Examples of these works include: Flora Fluminensis, by Frei José Mariano da Conceição Veloso (1742-1811), *Systema Materiae Medicae Vegetabilis Brasiliensis*, published in 1843, by Karl Friedrich Philipp Von Martius, Matéria Médica Brasileira, published between 1862 and 1864, by Manuel Freire Allemao Cysneros.

In the 20th century, the most important work on medicinal plants was Pio Correia's

Dicionârio das Plantas Ùteis do Brasil e das Exóticas Cultivadas, a six-volume collection published from 1926.

The 19th century was marked by the construction of anatomical and pathophysiological knowledge. The medical sciences moved away from herbalist knowledge and began to value symptomatology, supported by the theories of Clark, a biologist.

In 1805, morphine, an alkaloid from the poppy plant, was isolated for the first time and in 1838 salicin was extracted from the willow tree. From this, in 1860, the first drug was synthesized in the laboratory, aspirin. On the basis of this technique, there was a growing development of chemistry and new substances were isolated in the laboratory and new synthetic products emerged from them, leading to the gradual replacement of the use of plants by medicines produced in the laboratory, which occurred in full in the second half of the 20th century, motivated by several factors, one of the most important of which was the discovery of antibiotics.

Parallel to the replacement of the plant by medicine made from synthetic drugs, there has also been an intense effort to disqualify popular knowledge about medicinal plants, as evidenced by the ban on the practice of phytotherapy by lay people and even doctors in several countries.

This offensive against medicinal plants and popular knowledge was not restricted to the more developed countries, but spread to the colonies in America, Africa and Asia. For example, England banned the use of medicinal plants in India, which was unjustifiable given that this country, along with China, has the use of plants strongly rooted in its healing systems.

In the United States, in 1907, the government stopped subsidizing medical schools that taught the use of medicinal plants.

In Brazil, phytotherapy reached the 20th century as the most widely used therapy, despite the decline caused by the emergence of biological knowledge. This period was marked by economic prosperity driven by coffee growing, large-scale European immigration, increased urbanization, growing exports and the start of industrialization.

All this led to a worsening of the health situation in the cities, causing the emergence of major endemics and epidemics. In this new economic, health and scientific context, the use of plants was no longer appropriate.

During this period, all over the world, due to the accelerated construction of knowledge in the field of health, Biomedicine was strengthened as a medical rationality capable of guiding the understanding and handling of the health-disease process. In this biologicist model, there wasn't much room for the use of medicinal plants due to their link to popular knowledge. The scientific method was elevated to the category of the only way of constructing and applying true and effective knowledge. It was also the beginning of the pharmaceutical industry, with its promise of discoveries of medicines capable of combating all diseases and accessible to the entire population. This new situation favored the commodification of health, and the population's illness came to be seen as a source of profit.

In Brazil and around the world, phytotherapy has lost ground to synthetic medicines produced on a large scale. In short, the reasons that led to the decline in the use of medicinal plants throughout the 20th century were:

a) Scientific and technological development, with repercussions in the health sector;

b) The consolidation and expansion of the health professions, especially medicine, has led to a significant increase in the number of people with access to these professionals who did not use herbal medicine;

c) Combating the practice of healing by lay people, who normally used medicinal plants, on the part of health professionals and their representative bodies;

d) Disqualification of popular knowledge and exaltation of scientific knowledge as the only correct and reliable knowledge;

e) Development of the pharmaceutical industry and discovery of new drugs;

f) Practicality of using industrialized medicine;

g) Lack or insufficiency of studies proving the efficacy and safety of herbal medicines;

h) Lack of contact between the urban population and medicinal plants, leading to their devaluation;

i) The commodification of health.

Subsequently, we could see the gap between what was proposed and what was real. From the 1960s onwards, there began to be disenchantment with the promise of efficiency, safety and effectiveness of the medicalization of the population. Its efficacy was not enough to overcome diseases, since these are the result of multiple factors, including the lack of economic conditions that provide a healthy, quality life. What's more, the cost of synthetic medication makes it unaffordable for a large proportion of the population. These people have continued to use medicinal plants.

The disenchantment with synthetic medicine was part of the disenchantment with the technological and capitalist society that had created the expectation that technology would bring ease and abundance to everyone.

This led to the search for a natural lifestyle, a trend that was consolidated in the following decades, leading to the resurgence and strengthening of herbal medicine around the world.

Where herbal medicine has always been a widespread practice, this resurgence has been more intense, such as India and China. In this country, with the victory of the Communist Party, there was a great incentive to use medicinal plants, mainly through barefoot doctors. Traditional Chinese Medicine has herbal medicine as one of its main therapies, as does Ayurvedic Medicine (India). These conventional practices coexist on an equal footing with Biomedicine.

This growing trend has been seen all over the world. In Europe, in countries such as England, Germany and Spain, herbal medicines are widely consumed by a large part of the population. This growth can also be seen in universities, through teaching and research into medicinal plants.

In the United States, this growth is also taking place, but herbal medicines are marketed as food supplements.

Phytotherapy and other natural medicines and complementary practices can be used at the same time as allopathy, as a substitute for or complement to each other, depending on the nature of the illness, the patient's economic conditions, the structure of the health services and the training of health professionals.

The revival of herbal medicine in recent times has been due to a number of factors, such as scientific studies proving its efficacy, safety and effectiveness; easy access to plants; the population's belief in its efficacy and safety; the inclusion of herbal medicine in the population's cultural context; the use of medicinal plants through simple forms of preparation; belief in the low possibility of adverse effects, etc.

However, you need to know that the therapeutic action of medicinal plants and herbal medicines is based on the same principle as allopathic medicines, which is to cure through active ingredients that can also have adverse effects, which requires care. We need to overcome the myth that because plants are natural, they don't do any harm. When the correct dose, preparation and route are not used, the plant, even if it is medicinal, can cause problems for the individual, such as intoxication.

4 PHYTOTHERAPY IN THE UNIFIED HEALTH SYSTEM (SUS)

With the creation of the Unified Health System (SUS) in 1990, universal and comprehensive care was established. As a consequence, the multiple forms of treatment began to be valued. Within this new approach, herbal medicine has gained many followers among health professionals, managers and users of the SUS and among university professors and researchers.

Currently, primary care in the SUS is carried out mainly through the Family Health Program (PSF) teams that work in the Family Health Basic Units (UBSF).

These units are located in the communities themselves. Most of the illnesses treated by the PSF teams can be treated with herbal medicine. This highlights the importance of increasing the use of herbal medicine in the Unified Health System (SUS).

In 1988, therefore before the creation of the SUS, Resolution No. 08 of the Interinstitutional Planning and Coordination Commission (CIPLAN) regulated the implantation and implementation of herbal medicine in health services. However, the mere existence of the law was unable to bring this objective to fruition. However, despite the difficulties, phytotherapy and other natural medicines and complementary practices have grown considerably.

Reflecting this growth, on May 3, 2006, the Ministry of Health, through Ordinance 971, formulated the National Policy for Integrative and Complementary Practices (PNPIC) for the Unified Health System. Initially, this policy included phytotherapy, herbal medicine, traditional Chinese medicine (acupuncture) and thermalism.

The creation of this policy was very important as it establishes guidelines and measures for the implementation and development of the practices it covers. In the area of herbal medicine, the guidelines are:

1- Preparation of the National List of Medicinal Plants and the National List of Herbal Medicines;

2- Providing access to medicinal plants and herbal medicines for SUS users;

3- Training and continuing education for health professionals in medicinal plants and phytotherapy;

4- Monitoring and evaluation of the insertion and implementation of medicinal plants and phytotherapy in the SUS;

1- Strengthening and broadening popular participation and social control;

6- Establishment of a funding policy for the development of actions aimed at implementing medicinal plants and phytotherapy in the SUS;

7- Encouraging research and development of medicinal plants and herbal medicines, prioritizing the country's biodiversity;

8- Promoting the rational use of medicinal plants and herbal medicines in the SUS;

9- Guaranteed monitoring of the quality of herbal medicines by the National Health Surveillance System;

In order to make this policy operational, the Health Care Secretariat of the Ministry of Health published Ordinance No. 853, on 17/11/2007, which includes the practices contained in Ordinance 971 in the table of services/classifications of the National System of Health Establishments (SCNES), with code 068. This decree establishes the professionals who can carry out the practices that are part of the PNPIC in the SUS.

In addition, the National Policy for Medicinal Plants and Herbal Medicines was created by Presidential Decree No. 5813 of June 222, 2006. This policy has clear objectives and guidelines related to the themes and details the attributions of the various ministries and other public bodies so that it can actually be implemented in the Unified Health System.

Given the prospect of increasing phytotherapy in the SUS, Brazilian universities are faced with the challenge of introducing or increasing its teaching in undergraduate courses, as well as extension and research into medicinal plants.

The consolidation of herbal medicine in the SUS is justified for a number of reasons, such as: it provides health professionals with another form of treatment; the financial costs are lower; it has less potential to cause adverse effects; it is easy to access; the cultural inclusion of herbal medicine in people's habits and customs; it guarantees users the right to choose their preferred treatment; it facilitates popular participation in the SUS, rescuing popular knowledge; it is a source of employment and income.

However, many difficulties need to be overcome, such as: **the lack of knowledge and/or disbelief of some health professionals and managers; the insufficient number of professionals with knowledge of herbal medicine; the deficiency of herbal medicine teaching in undergraduate and specialization courses; the need for initial investment, such as the creation of laboratories to produce herbal medicine; the lack of knowledge about herbal medicine among the population**

or their misunderstanding of it, etc.

5 BASIC CONCEPTS IN HERBAL MEDICINE

Adjuvant: Substance of natural or synthetic origin added to the medicine with the aim of preventing alterations, correcting and/or improving the organoleptic, biopharmacotechnical and technological characteristics of the medicine.

Carminative: An agent that favors and causes the expulsion of intestinal gas. **Catarrhal**: A more energetic purgative than a laxative and less dratic.

Cholagogue: Agent/Substance that causes and favors the production of bile. **Choleretic**: Agent/Substance that increases the release of bile.

Derivatives of plant drugs: Products extracted from plant raw materials: extract, tincture, oil, wax, exudate, juice, etc.

Plant drug: Plant or its parts, after collection, stabilization and drying processes, which can be whole, shredded, crushed or pulverized.

Emmenagogue: Agent that restores menstrual flow.

Stomachic: An agent that stimulates the secretory activity of the stomach. **Ethnopharmacology:** Discipline that studies how traditional populations interact with plants and how they use them to treat their illnesses.

Herbal formula: Quantitative list of all the components of a herbal medicine.

Phytopharmaceutical: Medicinal product made from substances of plant origin, but in isolated form.

Herbal medicine: Medicinal product obtained using exclusively plant active raw materials. It is characterized by knowledge of the efficacy and risks of its use, as well as the reproducibility and consistency of its quality. Its efficacy and safety are validated through ethnopharmacological surveys of use, techno-scientific documentation in publications or phase 3 clinical trials.

A herbal medicine is not considered to be one whose composition includes isolated active substances of any origin, or associations of these with plant extracts.

Marker: Component or class of chemical compounds (e.g. alkaloids, flavonoids, fatty acids, etc.) present in the raw plant material, ideally the active ingredient itself, and preferably one that correlates with the therapeutic effect, which is used as a reference in the quality control of the raw plant material and herbal medicines.

Raw plant material: Fresh medicinal plant, plant drug and plant drug derivative.

Medicinal product: A pharmaceutical product, technically obtained or prepared, for prophylactic, curative, palliative or diagnostic purposes.

Complete official botanical nomenclature: Genus, species, variety, author of the binomial, family **Official botanical nomenclature**: Genus, species and author.

Botanical nomenclature: Genus and species.

Active ingredient of herbal medicine: Chemically characterized substance or chemical classes (e.g. alkaloids, flavonoids, fatty acids, etc.) whose pharmacological action is known and which is responsible, in whole or in part, for the therapeutic effects of the herbal medicine.

New herbal medicine: A **medicine** whose efficacy, safety and quality have been scientifically proven by the competent federal body at the time of registration, and which may serve as a reference for the registration of similar medicines.

Traditional herbal medicine: A **medicine** made from a medicinal plant, used in accordance with popular tradition, with no known or reported evidence of a risk to the user's health, whose efficacy has been validated through ethnopharmacological and usage surveys, technical-scientific documentation or indexed publications.

Similar herbal medicine: **A** medicine that contains the same plant raw materials, in the same concentration of active ingredient or markers, using the same route of administration, pharmaceutical form, dosage and therapeutic indication as a herbal medicine considered as a reference.

Medicinal plant - A plant species designated by its scientific and/or popular name and used for therapeutic purposes.

Active ingredient: Chemically characterized substance, or group of them, whose pharmacological action is known and which is responsible, in whole or in part, for the therapeutic effects of the herbal medicine.

Natural product: Any substance found in nature (vegetable, mineral or animal) of organic or inorganic origin that can be used directly or processed by humans.

6 POPULAR KNOWLEDGE AND SCIENTIFIC KNOWLEDGE

Phytotherapy is a field in which the question of popular knowledge and scientific knowledge is most often discussed. For a long time, all the information about medicinal plants came from popular knowledge, built up by observing the effect of plants on animal and human organisms and transmitted mainly through oral tradition.

With the consolidation of the various health professions and the increase in the number of professionals in this area, there was a strong movement to occupy all the spaces legally allocated to these professions and to do this it became necessary to remove all those who practiced the art of healing without having the legal qualification.

People who had always treated people's illnesses, many of them with great dedication and practical knowledge, came to be considered quacks. In order to exclude these people quickly and completely, their entire arsenal of knowledge and therapies came to be considered incorrect and ineffective. As a result, medicinal plants were relegated to the background, giving priority to the use of medicines made in laboratories and pharmaceutical industries, which were considered to be more effective and easier to use.

However, the expectations created by the development of the pharmaceutical industry have not been fully realized, causing a certain disenchantment in people, who have become interested in alternative therapies, especially herbal medicine.

The increase in the use of phytotherapy has forced academics to study and research medicinal plants, validating their efficacy and safety. But this was done by establishing a dichotomy between popular knowledge and scientific knowledge. The latter came to be seen as the guarantor of the safe use of plants. Scientific knowledge was seen as insufficient or even ineffective, perhaps even dangerous. In this way, it would be inadvisable to use plants based on indications from popular knowledge.

Science is not the only way to access knowledge and truth. Popular or vulgar knowledge, sometimes called common sense, is not distinguished from scientific knowledge either by its veracity or by the nature of the object known. What differentiates them is the form or method and the instruments of knowing.

Both common sense and science aim to be rational and objective. However, the ideal of rationality, understood as a coherent systematization of well-founded and verifiable statements, is achieved much more through the theories that make up the core of science than through common knowledge, understood as the accumulation of loosely linked parts or pieces of information. In turn, the ideal of objectivity, i.e. the construction of true and impersonal images of reality, cannot be achieved without going beyond the narrow confines of everyday life and private experience.

This is why common sense, or popular knowledge, can only achieve limited objectivity, just as its rationality is limited, because it is closely linked to perception and action. Despite its limited rationality and objectivity, we can say that popular knowledge is the common, ordinary and spontaneous way of knowing. We acquire it in direct contact with things and human beings. It is the knowledge that fills our daily lives and that we possess without having sought it out or studied it, without applying a method and without having reflected on it.

Its characteristics are that it is **superficial, sensitive, subjective, unsystematic and uncritical. However, like scientific knowledge, it is verifiable and fallible. It is also evaluative, reflexive and inaccurate when it seeks to generalize.** Despite its limitations, popular knowledge is useful and can and should be used by those who build knowledge within the scientific method. That's why there shouldn't be competition, but complementarity.

From this point of view, it is essential that those who work with medicinal plants, from a scientific point of view, seek out popular knowledge and pass on the information acquired through the scientific method to the agents who have it. Disqualifying information about medicinal plants that comes from the grassroots is a prejudiced attitude that is not committed to the reality in which we live and to building a fairer and more fraternal model of society.

7 PRECAUTIONS FOR THE PROPER USE OF MEDICINAL PLANTS

01ª - Knowing how to identify: Be very careful when you name a plant or get a recipe from a book where there is no drawing of the plant or its name in Latin. This is because the popular name varies from one region to another.

Give preference to fresh plants chosen correctly from the user's own cultivation sites. Dried plants should only be used when purchased from a responsible and safe source.

02a - Knowing which part of the plant to use: You need to know the plant and which parts are used: root, bark, leaves, whole plant, fruit and seeds.

03a - Know the toxicity of the plant: There are many plants that are toxic and many others that can be, depending on who takes it, how much they take and how they take it. **Children and the elderly are more easily intoxicated.** For this reason, much more care should be taken with the dose. Avoid taking teas during pregnancy. Many plants have an abortifacient and teratogenic effect (malformation of the child), such as quebra-pedra (*Phylanthus niruri* L.), capim santo (*Cymbopogon citratus* DC Stapf). Frequent use of tea by children who are breastfeeding should be avoided, as they may want to switch from milk to tea.

There are plants that, even in small quantities, are potentially poisonous, such as spirea (*Nerium oleander* L.) and nobody-can-eat-me (*Diffenbachia picta* Schot). It is advisable to be familiar with toxic plants.

04a - Know where to collect: Don't collect medicinal plants from the banks of rivers, polluted streams, sewers or roadsides because they are usually contaminated by car fumes, pesticides, etc. Nowadays, it's best to develop a community medicinal plant garden and then grow the basic plants of each area, according to the data research (ethnobotany) carried out beforehand.

05a - Knowing how to collect: When collecting leaves from a plant, don't remove all the leaves from a branch. It is through leaves that plants absorb the sun's rays. Discard leaves that are old, bitten by insects, moldy or otherwise contaminated.

The bark should be removed in small pieces, only from one side of the plant, as encircling the stem can cause death.

06ª - Know when to harvest: The best times to harvest are in the morning, just after the dew has completely dried, and in the late afternoon on sunny days. For aromatic plants, harvesting in the late afternoon is recommended, especially on very hot days, to avoid the evaporation of substances that are easily volatile under the action of the sun. There are differences in the time of harvest from one species to another; the ideal would be a plant collection calendar that indicates the right season, as with vegetables. For many plants, the right time to collect leaves is when the reproductive organs, such as those that form buds and flowers, begin to appear.

07a - Know how to dry and preserve: Flowers and leaves should be placed in the shade to dry in a ventilated, clean place in thin layers to prevent only the top ones from drying out. Three to five days is enough. Another method is to hang the flower branches and leaves on a clothesline until they dry. The bark should be scraped lightly and washed under running water to remove any dust, mud or insects from the surface and then placed in the sun to dry.

Roots should be washed and dried. In the case of very thick roots and husks, it is advisable to cut them into small, thin pieces after washing and lay them out to dry. Seeds should be harvested from ripe, healthy fruit, cleaned by sieving or washing and dried in the sun. These are the plant parts that last the longest.

When natural conditions of heat and wind are not available, drying can be done in an oven at a temperature of no more than 40° C. After drying, the plant parts should be reduced to small pieces, with the exception of the seeds, and stored in a clean, dry glass with a lid and protected from sunlight. A label with the name of the plant and the date of collection should be attached to the jar. It is advisable to always check for mold, insect contamination, etc., which will make them unfit for consumption. It is suggested that the stock be renewed every three to six months. **08a - Know how to prepare:** There are different methods of preparing herbal remedies. For example: infusion, decoction, maceration, etc. Avoid using iron, aluminum, copper or plastic pots; give preference to glass pots (which can be fired), porcelain or clay. It is also important to know how much of the plant to use in the preparation. Once prepared, medicines should be stored well. **09a - Knowing how to use:** Be careful when using plants. Observe whether the indication is for internal use (ingestion) or external use (local use). Many plants, such as comfrey (*Symphytum officinale* L.), should not be ingested, but only used in healing applications. You shouldn't mix many plants in the same medicine or take several of them at the same time.

10a - Knowing how much to use: It's important to know how much herbal medicine to take. You can't abuse the dosage. The popular saying "it's the big blow that kills the snake" should not be followed, as plants have adverse effects if they are used in high concentrations or for a long time.

In chronic diseases that require ongoing treatment, it is important to follow up with your doctor and laboratory. In these cases, the same plant should not be used for too long.

8 WAYS OF PREPARING AND USING MEDICINAL PLANTS

The effectiveness of herbal medicines depends on various factors, such as the way they are prepared and used. They can be prepared and used according to pharmaceutical techniques or using simpler techniques such as homemade preparations.

Simple ways to prepare it are:

CHA - Tea can be prepared as a decoction, infusion or macerate.

1- **Decoct** - A decoct is a preparation in which the active ingredients of plants are extracted in boiling water. It is used for roots, stems, bark and seeds. The part of the plant to be used must be thoroughly washed and cut and left to simmer for up to 15 minutes. Plants that have active ingredients that evaporate should not be used to make decoctions. For plants that contain a lot of tannin, the boiling time should be shorter.

2- **Infusion** - An infusion is a preparation that extracts the active ingredients from plants by pouring boiling water over the parts of the plant that have been washed, cut and placed in a container. After pouring in the water, the container is covered and left to stand for 15 minutes. The infusion is used for leaves, flowers and fruit.

3- **Macerate** - The macerate is prepared by placing the well-washed and finely chopped plant parts in a container of drinking water at room temperature for a period of 24 to 48 hours, depending on the consistency of the plant parts used.

To prepare the teas, one to five grams of the plant part is used for every 100 ml of water. After preparation, the tea should be filtered (strained) and placed in a clean container and consumed within 24 hours.

Teas used to treat colds, flu, bronchitis and fever should be sweetened and taken hot. Teas used for digestive ailments should be taken cold or iced, without sugar.

The dosage for tea is one cup, three times a day for adults. Children over 5 years old should take half a cup three times a day and children under 5 years old should take it individually.

Tea is the most common way of using medicinal plants because it is so easy to make, but it has the disadvantage of not being suitable for long-term preservation and it is difficult to quantify the raw plant material to be used.

Compound syrup - Compound syrup, made according to pharmaceutical standards, is prepared by adding 10ml of the tincture or alcohol and simple syrup in sufficient quantity to (qsp) complete 100 ml of compound syrup.

To make simple syrup, add 85 grams of sugar to 45 ml of distilled water and bring the mixture to a simmer. You have simple syrup. It is filtered and cooled. In this proportion, you should have 100 ml. If you don't have enough, add more water until you reach this volume. A chemical preservative (Nipagin) is added to the compound syrup, at a concentration of 0.02% w/v. The result is a 10% syrup, which must be packed in suitable packaging.

Homemade **lick** or syrup is prepared using 45 ml of the decoction, infusion or macerate for 85 g of sugar, or, to make it easier, twice the number of grams of sugar for the volume of tea. Example: for 50ml of tea, use 100 grams of sugar. This mixture should be brought to a simmer until molasses forms. When cold, the lick should be strained, topped up if necessary, placed in a clean container and stored properly.

This form is more suitable for making syrup from the decoction. When making tea to be made into a lick, you have to use ten times more vegetable raw material than when making tea to be taken as such. This is because the amount of syrup that is taken is much smaller than the amount of tea. In this way, the active ingredients in the two preparations remain the same.

Another homemade way of making the lick is to lay the leaves of the plants in layers, each covered with a little sugar and bring to a simmer. After a certain time, the water contained in the leaves mixes with the sugar to form molasses and the active ingredient is extracted. At the end, it is filtered and stored in a suitable container.

The dosage of the syrups is one tablespoon three times a day for adults. Children over the age of 5 should take half the dose and children under the age of 2 should be given an individual dose.

Tincture - To prepare the tincture, dry parts of the plants are used, well cut and bruised, which are placed in alcohol. In this case, 70% alcohol is used. To prepare 1 liter of tincture, 200 g of the plant are used and enough alcohol to cover the parts of the plant, leaving them to macerate for a period of 5 to 10 days. After this period, filter and top up with alcohol to 1 liter and store in a clean container away from light.

Alcohol - To prepare alcohol, use green parts of the plant, finely chopped or passed through a blender, and 95° alcohol. To prepare 1 liter of alcohol, 500 g of the plant and enough alcohol to cover the plant parts are used, leaving them to macerate for 5 to 10 days. After this period, the macerate is filtered (strained) and the volume is brought up to 1 liter with alcohol. Store in a clean container away from light.

This is the way to prepare tinctures and alcoholic drinks according to pharmaceutical standards. In popular circles, it is common to add water to alcohol when preparing tinctures and alcoholic drinks. This is not advisable as it compromises the extraction and preservation capacity.

The dosage for tinctures and alcoholic drinks is 30 drops, three times a day, which should be taken with a little water. Children over the age of five should take half the dose and children under the age of two should have their dosage individualized.

Ointment - The ointment can be prepared using 70% petroleum jelly and 30% lanolin. The lanolin and petroleum jelly should be melted over a low heat and when the mixture is cold, you have a simple ointment. It is advisable to leave it for a day.

For every 100 g of simple ointment, add 05 ml of tincture or alcohol and stir well to make the mixture homogeneous. This is how an ointment is prepared according to pharmaceutical techniques. In popular circles, there are various "recipes" for ointments using beeswax and paraffin.

Liquid **soap -** Liquid soap is prepared by placing 200g of coconut soap cut into small pieces in enough water to dissolve it. Place on a low heat until the soap is dissolved and homogenized. Then leave to stand.

From the part of the plant to be used, usually leaves, flowers, fruit and young twigs, use 200 grams and enough water to liquefy it in a blender. Filter and add to the liquid soap, topping up with water to 1 liter or approximately the same volume, depending on the consistency you want for the soap. Use it three or four times a day during the bath, leaving the body soapy for about 20 minutes.

Another variant of liquid soap is one in which the tincture and/or alcohol content of the plant(s) is added to the dissolved soap.

Soap - To make soap, use a glycerin base and the plant's tincture or alcohol. For every 100 grams of glycerin base, you need 5 to 10 ml of tincture or alcohol. First put the glycerine base on the fire to melt. Once this has happened, let it cool down a little and add the alcohol or tincture. The mixture is stirred well and placed in the mold to cool, from where the soap is removed when it is solid.

Powder - To prepare the powder, the part of the plant to be used must be dried well and crushed or ground. The powder is then sieved and stored in a clean, suitable container.

Juice - Juice is prepared by squeezing or crushing the leaves of the plant in a blender and then filtering them. The juice should be made at the time it is to be used.

Juice - To obtain the juice, pound the plant in a mortar and pestle or in a cloth until as much juice as possible comes out. If the plant has little water, you can add a little water and leave it to soak for an hour, then squeeze or pound it again. Finally, filter the liquid that comes out.

Salad - Some medicinal plants can be used in the form of salads. To make them, simply cut the plants into small pieces that should be eaten immediately.

Poultice **-** To make a poultice, the fresh plant is pounded into a paste which is placed directly on the affected area and can be covered with a cloth.

Cataplasm - To make a cataplasm, you proceed in the same way as you would to prepare a poultice, but to the paste you add some dough, such as flour, to make it more consistent.

Ointment - To make an ointment, use 100 g of vegetable fat and 5 to 10 ml of tincture or alcohol from the plant to be used. Put the vegetable fat on the fire until it melts.

Let it cool down a little and slowly add the tincture or alcohol, stirring the mixture well to homogenize it. Instead of tincture or alcohol, you can use the juice of the plant, extracted by crushing the leaves and stems (when fine and juicy).

Liniment - To make a liniment, use the juice of the plant's leaves mixed with a little oil. It is used to massage the affected area.

Compress - To make a compress, prepare a 5% decoction or infusion of the plant and soak a clean cloth in it and apply it to the affected area.

Bath - Make a 5% decoction or infusion of the plant and, after filtering, add it to the bath water. The bath should be taken slowly.

Mouthwash and gargle - Make a 5% decoction or infusion of the plant, filter it and then make a mouthwash and/or gargle.

Inhalation - For inhalation, use the 5% decoction or infusion, which should be placed in a glass while still hot. Use a piece of paper to make a funnel that fits into the glass, through which the steam produced is inhaled.

These are the forms of preparation and use of homemade medicines based on medicinal plants. As far as preparations according to pharmaceutical standards are concerned, in addition to the tincture, alcohol, ointment and syrup discussed here, there are many others such as elixir, extract, cream, gel, capsule, etc.

Dilution of alcohol - FRANCOUER'S formula: X = V. G'/G

X = volume of alcohol to be removed from the container to add the amount of distilled water needed to complete the volume. V = volume of final alcohol (after dilution) G' = grade of alcohol you want to obtain (final grade). G = grade of alcohol available.

Necessary precautions when preparing medicines with medicinal plants

Use filtered or boiled water;

Always wash your hands thoroughly;

Tie up your hair (caps if possible);

Make sure all utensils are properly cleaned;

Avoid talking near the preparation (wear masks if possible);

Use clean, scalded bottles;

Keeping the room where medicines are prepared clean.

9 CHEMICAL CONSTITUENTS OF MEDICINAL PLANTS

Plants synthesize chemical compounds from the nutrients and water extracted from the soil and the light they receive. Many of these compounds, or groups of them, can cause reactions in organisms. These are the active ingredients. Some of these substances can be toxic, depending on the dose used.

A medicinal plant is one that contains one or more active ingredients, giving it therapeutic activity.

When combining medicinal plants to prepare herbal medicines, their chemical composition must be observed so that they act synergistically. It is also important to remember that the dose is fundamental in some cases, as many substances can reverse the effect or even become toxic if the dose is increased.

The active principles of a plant are not always known, but it can still have satisfactory medicinal activity and be used, as long as it doesn't have acute or chronic toxic effects, which have already been verified by research, or even by popular knowledge in some cases.

In phytotherapy, the plant, or its parts, is used in its entirety, with all its chemical constituents, conferring therapeutic activity somewhat different from that presented by the isolated active ingredients, as there may be synergisms that favor the plant's pharmacological activity. These are called phytocomplexes.

Plants, in general, have a rich and varied range of active ingredients inside them. Some plants may have dozens of active ingredients, many of which interact with each other, which explains why certain plants act on various diseases.

Active ingredients can be divided into groups that have chemical and structural similarities. There are several groups of active ingredients. These are the result of secondary metabolism in plants. Primary metabolism produces substances necessary for growth, respiration and photosynthesis, such as amino acids, proteins, vitamins, carbohydrates, lipids, etc. Primary metabolites are widely distributed in plants. In secondary metabolism, the metabolites produced are restricted to certain plants and have a defense function, adaptation to the environment and biological competition.

Secondary Metabolism

Medicinal substances are produced by the plant and have very specific functions within the plant, as seen above. Most of the time, they are the result of secondary metabolism and therefore have a function linked to the plant's ecology, i.e. the plant's relationship with its environment.

Secondary metabolism differs from primary metabolism basically because it doesn't have reactions and products that are common to most plants, but is specific to certain groups. Respiration, for example, is part of primary metabolism. Secondary metabolites have certain characteristics, such as:

a) Not as vital to plants, in most cases, as alkaloids;

b) They are expressions of the chemical individuality of individuals and differ from species to species, both qualitatively and quantitatively;

c) They are produced in small quantities.

In addition, these substances can be present in the plant all the time or only produced by specific stimuli. Thus, the regulation of secondary metabolism depends on the plant's genetic capacity to respond to internal or external stimuli and the existence of these stimuli at the appropriate time.

Generally, plant species have more than one of these groups of substances. What usually differentiates medicinal plants is that the concentrations of these substances are higher, hence their use in therapy. Some genera and some plant families have very specific substances that can characterize them.

The Influence of the Environment on the Production of Active Ingredients

The concentration of active ingredients or drugs in the plant depends on genetic control (inherent capacity of the plant) and stimuli provided by the environment. Normally, these stimuli are characterized as "stress" situations, such as an excess or deficiency of some production factor for the plant. Once the plant is "competent" to produce drugs, its concentration of active substances can be altered by climatic and edaphic factors, exposure to microorganisms, insects, other herbivores and pollutants.

Among the climatic factors, temperature plays a very important role in plant survival, as it is most closely linked to plant growth and development. Species that are poorly adapted to the temperatures of a region will have serious problems in producing biomass and active ingredients, as this condition influences primary metabolism (respiration and photosynthesis) and, consequently, secondary metabolism. All other climatic factors are directly or indirectly related to temperature.

Light is also of great importance in photosynthetic processes and flower induction (photoperiod). Some plants, when exposed to direct sunlight, produce more coumarins, such as chambà or chachambà (*Justicia pectoralis*). In shade plants, this effect may be reversed.

Some plants need a certain number of hours of light per day (photoperiod) in order to flower. Thus, plants in tropical regions need a number of hours of light below a certain value (critical photoperiod) or they are insensitive, i.e. they can flower normally, regardless of this factor. Plants from temperate regions, on the other hand, usually need a longer photoperiod than the critical one for their species, such as lavender (*Lavandula officinalis*), which needs a photoperiod of more than 12 hours a day for three or four days.

The importance of this is mainly in determining when to harvest these species, as lavender has more essential oil at the start of flowering (in the flowering tops) and also in reproduction, as there may be a need to produce seeds, which is not possible without flowering and fertilization. Another aspect to consider in relation to the photoperiod is adjusting the planting time. Vegetative growth must be balanced with flowering, otherwise flower induction may occur earlier than desired, reducing the production of leaves and flowers.

Hydric stress (water deficiency in the soil) can promote increases in the concentration of active ingredients (essential oils and alkaloids). However, there can be a reduction in green mass production, which at certain limits can be disadvantageous. This is the case with vinegar (*Hibiscus sabdariffa*), whose ascorbic acid content in the leaves decreases under water deficit, as does biomass production.

In addition to climatic factors, edaphic factors (related to the soil) are also important.

Only a few chemical constituents will be covered here. These groups are not mutually exclusive, as they are separated either by physical characteristics, chemical properties or biological activity.

Organic Acids

They are found throughout the plant kingdom and can play important roles in the plant's primary metabolism (photosynthesis and respiration). Malic, citric, tartaric and oxalic acids are the most common. Others, such as ferric acid, may be less common. Tartaric acid and its salts can have a mild laxative action. Citric and tartaric acids can increase the flow of saliva (sialagogue), helping to reduce the number of bacteria that cause tooth decay.

In general, acids are laxatives, diuretics, stimulants of cellular respiration and metabolism. They are antioxidants and tissue regenerators. Oxalic acid and its potassium and calcium salts can stimulate the appearance of kidney stones and reduce the proportion of calcium in the blood, which can affect the functioning of the heart. Therefore, plants with a lot of oxalic acid or oxalate, such as monkey cane (*Costus sp.*), should not be used for long periods.

Alkaloids

Most of them have alkaline properties, due to the presence of amino nitrogen. They are the most diverse group of natural products. Essentially, they have only one thing in common, which is that they have at least one nitrogen atom in their structure. All alkaloids have N, C and H. They can be solid or liquid, colorless or yellow or purple.

In the plant cell, they are produced in the endoplasmic reticulum and are stored in the vacuoles of epidermal and hypodermal cells and lactiferous vessels. When in the form of salts, they are found in cell walls. They are present in leaves, seeds, roots and stems.

Their concentration can vary greatly during the year and may, at certain times, be restricted to certain organs. Plants from warm and tropical regions are richer in alkaloids than plants from cold regions. In general, their proportion is between 0.3 and 1%. In some cases, it can reach up to 10% of the plant's dry weight. They are usually more concentrated in the growing or forming parts (vegetative points). They give plants a bitter taste. However, not every plant that tastes bitter is due to the presence of alkaloids.

Only 10 to 15% of known plants have alkaloids in their composition. They predominate in angiosperms. In the papaveraceae family (poppies), all species contain these substances.

The names of alkaloids are often derived from the species from which they were isolated, such as the nicotine found in tobacco (*Nicotina tabacum*). They are divided into 15 groups according to their biochemical origin or structural similarity.

In the human body, they act on the central nervous system (calming, sedative, stimulating, anesthetic and analgesic). Morphine extracted from the poppy (*Papaver somniferum*) is an anesthetic. Caffeine, from coffee and guarana, is a stimulant. Hyoscyamine, found in the trumpet tree (*Datura stramonium*), is an example of an analgesic. Other alkaloids that can be toxic can also be found in the trumpet tree, the antidote to which is another alkaloid from a Brazilian plant, pilocarpine, found in Jaborandi (*Pilocarpus microphilus*), used to treat glaucoma.

Some alkaloids can be carcinogenic and others anti-tumor. The pyrrolizidine alkaloids found in comfrey (*Symphytum officinal* L.) are examples of cancer-causing alkaloids. Vincristine present in a plant called good night (*Chantarantus roseus)* is an example of an alkaloid with antitumor action. Of the 60 or so alkaloids present in nightshade, vincristine and vinblastine stand out for their use against some types of leukemia.

In general, plants with alkaloids can be toxic if used in larger quantities or inappropriately. Alkaloids were the first active ingredients isolated from plants. In 1803, the German Sertarmer isolated morphine.

Phenolic compounds

Phenol is one of the most important plant constituents and gives rise to several others, such as tannins. Salicylic acid, which is found in various plants and has antiseptic, analgesic and anti-inflammatory properties, is used in allopathic medicine in the form of a derivative, acetylsalicylic acid.

Inorganic compounds

They are normal constituents of plants that form the ash or residue after the organic matter has been removed. The most important are calcium and potassium salts. Potassium salts have diuretic properties, especially if they are accompanied by saponins and flavonoids, with the ability to eliminate sodium from the body along with water, as well as expelling residual substances accumulated in the bloodstream.

Calcium salts contribute to the formation of bone structure and the regulation of the nervous system and heart, giving the patient greater resistance to infections. Silicon salts are important for strengthening connective tissues, especially in the lungs. It increases resistance to tuberculosis and strengthens nails, skin and hair.

The diuretic effect attributed to some plants with a high amount of silicon is usually due to the presence of flavonoids and saponins. Potassium salts are very soluble in water, which is why many teas have diuretic properties. Monkey cane (*Costus sp.*), for example, is very rich in potassium, which makes it an excellent diuretic. Calcium salts are usually not very soluble and are therefore not very extracted in teas. Silicon salts are only extracted by prolonged boiling. Normally, a balanced diet provides these minerals in the necessary quantities, and there is no need for herbal medicines.

Glycosides or Heterosides

They are substances formed by the combination of a reducing sugar called glycone and a non-sugar group called aglycone or genin. The latter is responsible for the therapeutic action. They taste bitter. There are various types of glycosides such as cardioactive, alcoholic, cyanogenetic, anthraquinonic, flavonoid, saponinic, coumarinic, etc.

Quinones

They are products of the oxidation of phenols. They are found in bacteria, fungi, lichens, gymnosperms and angiosperms and even in some animals, such as some arthropods and sea urchins. More than 1,500 types are known. The most important are naphthoquinones and anthraquinones.

They have a purgative action because they stimulate the peristaltic movements of the intestines 8-12 hours after ingestion. Their purgative action is also due to the fact that they reduce the absorption of water by the intestinal villi, leading to softening of the stools. Plants containing them should not be used orally, as they have a nephrotoxic action, leading to fluid retention.

Continued use of quinone-based laxatives can lead to inflammatory and degenerative processes and a severe reduction in peristalsis and even atony of the intestine, as well as a loss of electrolytes. The most common anthraquinone is aloin, found in *aloe vera*. Lapachol, from the purple ipe (*Tabebuia avelanedae*), is an example of a naphthoquinone. In addition to their laxative action, quinones have antibacterial, antifungal and antitumor effects.

Coumarins

It is a heteroside that has several basic forms: hydroxycoumarin, furanocoumarin, pyranocoumarin and dicoumarols. They can occur in leaves, fruits, seeds and roots. Coumarins can have an odor that characterizes a plant, as is the case with chachambà (*Justicia pectoralis*). One of the metabolites of coumarins, obtained by fermentation, is dicumarol, a powerful anticoagulant because it blocks the action of vitamin K. It is used in allopathy as the basis for drugs against thrombosis, in small doses, and as a poison for rats, in large doses. This is why plants rich in coumarins should be dried with care.

Coumarins also have an antimicrobial action and have been used since ancient times to treat skin diseases such as psoriasis, vitiligo, leucoderma, mycoses, dermatitis and eczema. Some coumarins, especially furanocoumarins (found in fig leaves, for example), can sensitize the skin under the action of ultraviolet rays, causing phytophotodermatitis (blisters, hyperpigmentation, erythema and blistering). Others, because of this property, are used to treat vitiligo by stimulating skin pigmentation. They are most commonly found in angiosperms.

Saponins

They are also heterosides. Their outstanding characteristic is that they foam when placed in water. They are used to synthesize cortisone (an anti-inflammatory drug) and sex hormones. Dioscin, extracted from a species of yam (carà), is hydrolyzed to release diosgenin, which is the raw material used in the synthesis of steroid hormones. The body can use them as precursors for other useful substances.

High concentrations of saponins in the bloodstream can be dangerous, as they can cause hemolysis due to the disorganization of red blood cell membranes. Fortunately, their absorption from the gastrointestinal tract is low, reducing the risk of poisoning when used orally.

In the intestine, they act by facilitating the absorption of certain substances, medicines or foods, by increasing the permeability of the membranes. This is the case with increased absorption of calcium and silicon.

They are mild laxatives, diuretics, digestives, anti-inflammatories and expectorants. They have an irritant effect on the mucous membranes of the digestive tract, causing vomiting, colic and diarrhea. The fact that saponins aid in the absorption of certain medicines means that plants containing them can be used in combination with others in teas. An example of the presence of saponins is in the juazeiro (*Zizyphus joazeiro* Mart) and beet ( ), whose juice is expectorant. Prolonged boiling can reduce or destroy the effectiveness of saponins and other heterosides.

Flavonoids

They are heterosides with 15 carbons. The term flavonoid comes from the Latin *flavus*, meaning yellow, because of the color they give to flowers. They can be colored or colorless. Flavonoids are more concentrated in the aerial part of plants, occurring to a lesser extent in roots and rhizomes.

They are very widespread secondary metabolites in the plant kingdom. Their biological function in plants is related to the attraction of pollinating insects and protection against harmful ones, reaction against viral and fungal infections, collaboration with hormones in the growth process, inhibition of enzymatic actions and participation in the redox systems of cells. Medicinally, they strengthen capillaries, such as rutin, found in rue (*Ruta graveolens* L.) and hesperidin, found in orange peel.

They are antisclerotic and anti-edematous (rutin and oxyethylrutin), coronary dilators (proanthocyanidins), spasmolytic and anti-hepatotoxic (silymarin), choleretic, diuretic, antimicrobial and anti-inflammatory (artemetin).

The great advantage of flavonoids or bioflavonoids (produced by plants) is their extremely low toxicity. They are essential for the complete absorption of vitamin C and normally occur wherever vitamin C is present. A balanced diet provides the necessary amount of flavonoids.

Cardioactive Glycosides

Exclusive to angiosperms where they are present in some genera and families. They are substances that are absorbed cumulatively by the body and can cause chronic intoxication. Their use in the treatment of heart disease is restricted to drugs extracted and purified on medical advice, since there is no way of adequately controlling the quantity of these substances ingested in the form of teas or other substances.

Digitoxin, found in foxglove (*Digitalis lanata and Digitalis purpurea*), is the most important glycoside in this group. A dose of around 10 mg can be lethal for a person weighing 70 kg. However, in small quantities it increases the heart's ability to contract. Although this effect was only described by Whitering in 1775, the use of *digitalis purpurea* as a cardiotonic dates back to the 12th century and it remains the main source of cardioactive glycosides.

They stimulate cardiac contractility and diuresis. They regulate electrical conduction and have a bradycardic effect.

Cyanogenetic glycosides

By hydrolysis, they release cyanide or prussic acid. The cyanide acid released in the stomach by the action of gastric juice blocks cytochrome oxidase, causing death by anoxia. An example of this glycoside is the linimarin present in the outer part of cassava (*Manihot esculenta* Grantz). Hence the need to remove the peel from the root before using it. Cassava roots are ground in the presence of heat, before being eaten, due to the ease with which cyanidic acid is inactivated when subjected to heat.

The roots can also be scalded and the water resulting from the first boiling should be thrown away. Most mammals have enzyme systems that inactivate cyanide, which means that a large intake is necessary for poisoning to occur.

Mucilages

Chemically, mucilages are complex polymers of acidic or neutral polysaccharides with a high molecular weight. All plants produce them and they are metabolized for growth and reproduction or stored as nutritional reserves.

These carbohydrates also have the following functions in the plant: water retention in the parenchyma of succulent plants; lubrication for the growth of root apices; adhesion to disperse some types of seeds and capture insects by carnivorous plants, regulation of the germination process of seeds and, possibly, protection against herbivores.

Mucilage can be found in seeds, stems, leaves and roots. Mucilage secretion can occur in various cell structures. Mucilage has the property, in aqueous solution, of producing a plastic or viscous mass, which is responsible for the laxative effect, as the water is retained in the intestine, preventing its contents from hardening. It also acts as a lubricant and, at the same time, increases the volume inside the intestine, stimulating its peristaltic movements.

All mucilages act on the mucous membranes.

Mucilages form a viscous film that covers the walls of the organs in the alimentary canal, helping to reduce irritation by acids and salts on inflamed or diseased areas, a property that plays an important role in cases of diarrhea, especially those caused by certain bacteria or irritating substances.

They are also very effective in cases of coughs caused by irritation of the mucous membranes of the respiratory tract and help to increase the secretion of mucus. An example of this activity is found in spearmint (*Plectrantus amboinicus* Lour.). Plants rich in mucilage are widely used in hot compresses, due to their ability to retain heat and the large amount of water, which allows the heat to gradually penetrate the tissues. They are also vulnerable and hemostatic, hence their use in skin wounds and gastric ulcers.

In small doses, mucilages reduce peristaltic movements and have an antidiarrheal action, while in larger doses the opposite occurs. When subjected to prolonged boiling, mucilages are degraded into sugars, reducing or eliminating their therapeutic activity. They have an antitussive and laxative action, reduce stomach acidity and produce a feeling of fullness.

Essential oils

They are volatile organic substances, well known for the smell that characterizes certain plants, such as menthol in mint, the eucalyptus smell given off by eucalyptol, etc. The aroma of plants containing essential oils is the result of the combination of their various fractions.

Resins differ from oils in that they contain both volatile and non-volatile substances of high molecular weight. Resins are the result of the oxidation and polymerization of essential oils and are not very water-soluble.

They can be found in a single plant organ or throughout the plant, where they act by attracting pollinating insects or warding off harmful insects, regulating transpiration and intervening with hormones in pollination. They are produced by various cellular structures.

The large number and diversity of substances included in this group of active ingredients is what determines the wide variety of pharmacological actions. The properties of oils are varied: antiviral, antispasmodic, analgesic, bactericidal, healing, expectorant, relaxing, vermifuge, etc. The menthol in mint (*Mentha piperita*) has an expectorant and antiseptic action; the thymol and carvacrol found in spearmint (Plectrantus amboinicus Lour) and pepper rosemary (*Lippia sidoides*) are antiseptic; eugenol from cloves (*Eugenia Coryophyllata* Thamb) is a local anesthetic and analgesic; and ascaridol, found in St. Mary's wort (*Chenopodium ambrosioides*), is a vermifuge.

In some cases, essential oils can even increase the production of white blood cells. Certain essential oils act by increasing the secretions of the digestive system, which justifies their use as digestives. Others are expectorants, as they stimulate bronchial secretion, such as eucalyptol. Substances such as eucalyptol and menthol, which are eliminated by the pulmonary and urinary tracts, are considered to be antiseptics of the respective systems. In general, high doses of essential oils can cause nephritis and hematuria.

They are easily transported by the body and can cross the placenta, as well as reaching breast milk. It is recommended that plants containing them receive special attention when harvesting, drying and, above all, storing them, which should be done in well-sealed containers to avoid further losses. Some essential oils can be used to control diseases and pests of medicinal plants, given the bactericidal, bacteriostatic, fungicidal and insecticidal action of some substances.

Bitter substances

They are a group of compounds with no chemical similarity between them, having in common only a bitter taste and therapeutic activity. They belong to various chemical groups. In general, bitter compounds stimulate the functioning of the glands, producing various effects, such as increased secretion of digestive juices, whetting the appetite (aperient). The activity of the liver can be especially stimulated, increasing the production and flow of bile (*Plectrantus barbatus*).

The effect of these compounds is very variable, because in some cases, if taken before meals, in small quantities, they are strong appetizers, but if the dose is increased, there is a reduction in appetite, while a slightly higher dose restores the lost appetite. Some compounds also have diuretic, antibiotic, antifungal and antitumor activities. In the cotton plant (*Gossypium hirsutum*), there is a bitter principle with male contraceptive activity, as it reduces the amount of sperm. Some characteristic examples of these compounds are: absinthe in wormwood (*Artemisia absinthium*), cynicin in holy thistle (*Cnicus benedictus*), cynarin in artichoke (*Cynara scolymus*).

Tannins

They are complex, polyphenolic chemical substances linked to other aromatic compounds, which are distributed in all parts of the plant to protect it against herbivores, inhibit seed germination and the action of nitrogen-fixing bacteria, etc. Their presence in plants is easily perceived by the astringency of chewing a part containing them, such as a green guava. They are most concentrated in the roots and bark and in smaller quantities in the leaves and fruit.

They have the property of precipitating proteins and are responsible for tanning hides and skins. In large doses, they can irritate mucous membranes. In small doses, they can make them impermeable, as they precipitate small amounts of proteins, which can prevent the penetration of harmful agents into damaged mucous membranes, facilitating, for example, the healing of burns, which also explains their anti-diarrheal property. Tannins thus help to form a protective layer on the skin and mucous membranes. They cause capillaries to contract and stop bleeding. Tannins can react with air and become inactive, and can also be destroyed by prolonged boiling of water.

They have antiseptic, anti-haemorrhagic, wound-healing and anti-diarrheal properties. There are three hypotheses for the antiseptic action of tannins: tannins inhibit the enzymes of bacteria and/or react with the substrates of these enzymes;

Tannins act on the membranes of microorganisms, modifying their metabolism; they react with metal ions, reducing their availability for the metabolism of these microorganisms.

10 HANDLING MEDICINAL PLANTS: BASICS OF CULTIVATION, COLLECTION, DRYING AND STORAGE.

Cultivation

The correct cultivation of medicinal plants is of fundamental importance for improving the production and quality of the raw plant material, guaranteeing its phytochemical and pharmacological quality.

In northeastern Brazil, we find a great diversity of ecosystems rich in medicinal plants, but they are largely devastated and many species, such as the purple Ipe (*Tabebuia avellanedae*), are threatened with extinction. On the other hand, extractive collection, as well as driving medicinal species to extinction, does not guarantee the phytochemical homogeneity of the harvested material when compared to plants grown under suitable agricultural conditions.

Before growing any medicinal species, we must be sure of its identification so that we don't make a mistake and grow the wrong plant. To do this, we should look for people who have knowledge of the subject.

Growing medicinal plants requires several precautions to ensure the quality of the raw material. The growing site should be close to a source of water such as a stream, well or tap. It should be protected from strong winds, receive sunlight throughout the day, depending on the species to be grown, and be located away from contaminated sites such as cesspits, animal husbandry, garbage, contaminated watercourses, roadsides, etc.

Once the site has been chosen, the ground needs to be cleared of all weeds, stones, stumps and glass. The beds should be fertilized with organic compost, such as well-decomposed plants, leaves, paper, manure and others, which can be prepared in an adjacent area. The manure (ox, chicken, pig) must be well tanned. Fresh manure ends up decomposing in the soil and thus steals nitrogen, which should only feed the plants. Fresh manure increases the temperature of the soil and can suffocate the roots of seedlings. In addition, substances contained in animal urine weaken plants and turn them yellow.

The soil in the bed should be turned over using a hoe or equivalent tool to a depth of 30 centimeters. The recommended size of the bed is 1 meter wide, 20 to 30 centimeters high and around 5 meters long. These measurements can be altered depending on the size of the plot and the type and quantity of plants to be grown.

The width of 1 meter makes it easier to work, as you can reach the seedlings in the center with your hands from either side. The length of 5 meters makes it easier to work all around the bed.

The height (20 to 30 centimeters) prevents waterlogging and the round measurements make it easier to calculate the amount of fertilizer and seeds to be placed per square meter. The spacing between the beds should be 30 to 40 centimeters, to make it easier to move between them. The surface of the bed should be level.

When possible, the soil should be analyzed and corrected if necessary.

It is important to lay out the length of the bed in a north-south direction. This way, the bed will receive an equal amount of sunlight over its entire area. The edges of the bed should be on a slope so that the water runs off easily. This way, the bed never gets waterlogged, which would damage production. Excess moisture leads to root rot and the appearance of fungi, which love warm, humid environments.

The furrows are small trenches that should be made along the length of the bed. The spacing between the furrows and their depth should be as indicated for each medicinal plant.

In addition to beds, which are more commonly used to grow small plants, you can also use pits for larger plants. These should be prepared at least 18 days before planting and spaced according to the medicinal plant to be planted. They should be 30 x 30 cm wide and 30 cm deep, on average.

The hole should be dug taking care to separate the top soil, which is about half the depth of the hole, from the bottom soil. The topsoil, which is fertile, can be mixed with organic fertilizer and put back in the hole, leaving it at a lower level than the soil, while the bottomsoil should be placed around it in a circular pattern to avoid flooding.

The soil in the beds, pits or seedbeds must not be too clayey. Excessively clayey soil retains too much moisture because it is difficult for water to pass through the pores of the soil. Excessive humidity not only encourages the appearance of diseases, but can also suffocate the roots of the seedlings.

Soil that is too clayey can crack during a drought and break off the roots. To make it less clayey, sand should be added to the right extent, until it becomes sandy-clay. This makes better use of irrigation water, which infiltrates more easily. Also make sure that the soil is very fine, without clods.

Soil that is too sandy (too loose, crumbly) is also harmful. Water runs off too easily, without the roots of the seedlings having time to absorb it. This makes the plant thirsty, altering the assimilation of nutrients, as water is the agent that dissolves them, making them assimilable by the roots.

Not all plants can be planted directly in the beds. In this case, we use seedbeds, which are places where seedlings are formed and then transplanted to their final location. You can use wooden crates, perforated basins, plastic bags, small beds or make them out of masonry. The boxes should have a few holes in the bottom to drain the water.

The soil in the seedbed must be loose, clean, well fertilized and kept constantly moist because it will serve as a bed for the seeds to germinate.

Sow at least one week after preparing the seedbed. Sowing can be done in a furrow or in a row.

Spread the seed over the seedbed, taking care to ensure even distribution. In a row, the furrows should be 01 cm deep (approximately 01 finger), at a distance of 10 cm (approximately half a palm) from each other. Once the seeds have been sown, they should be covered by sieving a thin layer of soil (from the bed itself) over the seeds. The seedbed should be covered with grass or straw. Water with a watering can in the morning and afternoon.

As soon as the seeds germinate, remove the straw or grass and build a pyre with a height of 2 meters, which should be covered with grass, straw or leaves to prevent the direct sunlight from burning the seedlings. Gradually remove the cover from the pyre when the leaves start to grow, to get them used to the sun. After a few days, the cover can be removed.

When the seedlings have at least 5 leaves or are 20 centimeters tall, they should be transplanted to their final location, the beds or pits. In the final location, the plants should be watered with an adequate amount of water. Too little water hinders plant growth and the dissolution of nutrients in the soil. Too much water causes these nutrients to be carried away, the roots to rot and organisms harmful to the plants to proliferate.

Watering should preferably be done in the morning and evening. To save water, especially where it is scarce, drip irrigation can be used, using plastic bottles with a small hole in the lid, placing the bottle in an inverted position.

The soil must be cleaned constantly and if it is done with a hoe or similar tool, care must be taken not to damage the roots. It is important to remove dry or diseased leaves and branches from the plants with a sharp-edged object such as knives or scissors.

The weeds removed when clearing the land should be placed around the trunk of the plant to keep the soil moist, provide the plant with nutrients and encourage the development of microfauna, which decompose the organic material and make holes in the soil, improving its aeration.

For the proper production of active ingredients, there must be a variety of plants in the same bed, forcing biological competition.

Pest control can be achieved through correct crop management, by planting plants in and around the bed that scare away insects, usually plants with strong smells, such as Holy Grass (*Cibopogum citratus*), Pepper Rosemary (*Lipia sidoides*), Rue (*Ruta graveolens*), and by using pesticides made from plants such as tobacco.

Collection

When collecting, we need to pay attention to various factors that interfere with the greater or lesser amount of active ingredients, such as the stage of development of the plant, the organ of the plant, the time of year and the time of day.

As for the parts of the plant, the general recommendations for harvesting them are as follows: the bark and inter-bark should be harvested when the plant has already set flower. Flowers, when flowering begins. Fruits and seeds should be picked when ripe. As for the roots, they should be harvested when the plant is mature and the stems and leaves, before the plant sets flowers. Ideally, however, each plant should have conclusive studies on the best time to harvest it.

In order to obtain good quality raw materials, certain precautions must be taken.

Regarding the health of the plant and its phytochemical quality: don't pick plants that are old or diseased, eaten by insects or with insect eggs. Don't pick plants from contaminated places. Pick the plant when it is mature and alive. When collecting specific parts, know the right age and time for collecting them.

As for the right time: don't pick the plants on rainy days, when they are wet with dew or in bright sunshine. Preferably harvest early in the morning or late in the evening.

As for preserving the species: don't remove all the leaves from a branch. In the case of bark, it is recommended to remove small pieces only from one side of the plant at a time. If you remove large pieces from around the trunk, you could cause the plant to die. When collecting plants in a public place or in an extractive way, always leave a few plants of each species so that they can grow and multiply.

With regard to accommodating the collected plants: for collection, use baskets or cardboard boxes, taking care not to pile the plants up or crush them, and take the collected plants as quickly as possible to dry, without letting them "heat up or darken".

Drying

Most medicinal plants are sold in dried form, making the drying process essential for the quality of the raw plant material.

Drying is important to prevent the material from spoiling, as the reduction in water content hinders the action of enzymes that inactivate the active ingredients and the proliferation of microorganisms.

Drying, due to the evaporation of the water contained in the cells and tissues of plants, reduces the weight of the material. For this reason, it promotes an increase in the percentage of active ingredients in relation to the weight of the material. When a plant is dried, its leaves lose 20 to 75% of their weight. The bark loses 45 to 65%. The roots lose 25 to 80% and the flowers generally lose between 15% and 80%.

Drying can be carried out under ambient conditions (natural drying) or with the use of ovens or dryers, etc. (artificial drying).

Natural drying is a slow process. This process, for domestic use, is recommended for regions with favorable climatic conditions, such as: good ventilation, low relative humidity and high temperatures.

Important precautions for natural drying:

As for when to start drying: drying should be started immediately after collection, because when the plants are collected, their enzymes come into play and modify the molecules of the active ingredients, which can make them inactive. Hence the need to stabilize the active ingredients

Cleaning the parts of the plant: the roots, bark and leaves should be washed. However, if they contain essential oils, they should be washed lightly. Ideally, wash the plant one or two days before collecting it. Flowers should not be washed.

As for the drying area: it must be clean, free from dust, insects and animals, with good ventilation.

As for exposure to the sun: in general, plants should be dried in the shade. In the case of bark and roots that have been washed and have absorbed water, they can be left in the sun for a while.

As for handling during drying: the plants should be dried separately and identified; in containers that allow good aeration; cut into small pieces; arranged in thin layers, which should be turned frequently to speed up drying.

In small herbal medicine production workshops, natural drying takes place in a specific room, where the various parts of the plants are placed on wire mesh trays in mesh cages with smaller holes to prevent insects from landing on the plant. Incandescent lights are placed on the trays to increase the temperature and reduce the humidity.

Artificial drying can be done using various methods. We will only talk about hot air drying here. Hot air drying is the process most commonly used for drying solids, provided they are heat-resistant.

The devices generally used are air circulating ovens. The temperature used ranges from 35 - 45°C. Temperatures above 45°C damage the plant organs and their contents, as they cause the plants to cook rather than dry, although they inactivate larger quantities of enzymes.

The drying time, whether natural or artificial, varies according to each plant and the part of the plant, due to the greater or lesser amount of water inside.

Storage

Medicinal plants must be stored correctly. Otherwise, they may spoil or alter their active ingredients. The plant should only be stored when it is very dry so that fungi (mold) and other microorganisms do not proliferate.

At this point, it is necessary to check all the material to be stored, discarding anything that is damaged or does not appear to be in good condition. To be stored, the plants should be reduced to smaller pieces so that they fit better in the container, which should be very clean.

Plants should preferably be kept in glass and in cool, ventilated places, out of direct sunlight.

You shouldn't store more than one plant in a single container, even for short periods of time. On the container in which you store the plant, you should write the name of the plant, the part of the plant and the date of storage.

The plant's shelf life depends on good collection and proper drying and storage, ranging from six months to a year. However, if possible, the stock of plants should always be renewed.

11 MEDICINAL PLANTS WITH ANTIMICROBIAL PROPERTIES

ROSEMARY

Scientific name: *Rosmarinum officinalis L.*

Family: *Labiatae.*

Popular names: rosemary, romero, garden rosemary, rosemary, rosemary tree.

Chemical composition:

Essential oil (0.5 to 2.0%): Alpha pinene* (25%), beta pinene*, camphene*, limolene, 1,8 cineol* (12%) and, above all, camphor, which accounts for 10 to 20% of the total essential oil.

Flavonoids: Diosmin, diosmetin, hispiludin, apigenin.

Terpenoids: Carnasol and ursolic acid.

Phenolic acids: caffeic, chlorogenic and rosmarinic **acids**.

It has antibacterial and antifungal activity. It is effective against *Staphylococus aureus, Staphylococus albus, Escherichia coli, Vibrio colerae and Candida albicans*. Carnasol and ursolic acid inhibited various microorganisms (*Staphylococus aureus, Escherichia coli, Lactobacillus brevis, Pseudomonas*, etc.) in spoiled foods . Rosmarinic acid and diosmin have anti-flammatory and antioxidant activity. Essential oils (especially cineole) have spasmolytic and analgesic activity.

Its oil is listed in several pharmacopoeias.

It is used as a food flavoring.

Indications: Antimicrobial, anti-inflammatory, spasmolytic, carminative.

Used parts: Leaves and branches.

How to use: It is used in the form of tea, alcohol and oil, extracted by steam.

Adverse and/or toxic effects: May cause erythema and dermatitis in sensitive people. High camphor content may cause epileptic seizures. May cause irritation of the renal endothelium.

Contraindications: Sensitive individuals, pregnancy (may cause miscarriage), breastfeeding and patients prone to seizures.

GARLIC

Scientific name: *Allium sativum* L.

Family: *Liliaceae*

Popular names: Garlic, common garlic, leek.

Chemical composition: Its essential oil contains around 50 volatile chemical components, all organic derivatives of sulphur, the main ones being allicin*, alliin* and ajoene.

Alkyne and other sulphur compounds in garlic are derived from alliin when it is degraded by the enzyme alliinase. Alliin and alliinase are separated in bulb cells. When garlic is bruised, the transformation process begins. The sulphur compounds in garlic degrade more slowly in an acidic environment, hence their greater effectiveness when taken with citrus fruit juice.

Pre-clinical, clinical and epidemiological studies show that garlic has remarkable antimicrobial properties: antibacterial, antiviral, antimycotic, antiprotozoal and antiparasitic.

Some types of bacteria sensitive to garlic are *Staphylococus, Helicobacter pylory, Escherichia, Proteus, Salmonella, Citrobacter, Klebisiella, Vibrio, Bacillus*, etc. Garlic inhibits the growth of 30 strains *of Mycobacterium*, made up of 17 species, including *Mycobacterium tuberculosis.*

Allicin destroys the thiol groups (-SH) that are essential for bacteria to proliferate.

It is hypothesized that garlic inhibits the growth of bacterial cells by first inhibiting RNA synthesis.

Garlic also has a range of activities against fungi such as *Mycrosporum, Ephydermophyton, Tricophyton, Candida*, etc.

In studies with garlic extract, it proved to be more effective than nystatin in the treatment of yeasts, including *Candida albicans*. In this case, garlic inhibits lipid synthesis. *In in vitro* studies, garlic has shown great activity against *Influenza* B, *Parainfluenza* type 3 and *Herpes simplex* type 1.

Indications: Antibacterial (various types of infections), antiviral, antimycotic, anticoagulant, vermifuge, hypolipidemic, antihypertensive, etc.

Part used: Bulb

Directions for use: Adults - Take 2 to 4 ml of garlic tincture (made in a 1:5 ratio in 45% alcohol) diluted in a little water, 3 times a day. It is best used *fresh.* In this case, you should eat 4 g of raw garlic a day with food.

Adverse and/or toxic effects: Allicin is reasonably toxic and an irritant to the stomach. It is responsible for the characteristic smell of garlic. In high doses, it can cause headaches, burning in the gastrointestinal tract, nausea, vomiting, diarrhea, kidney problems and dizziness.

Contraindications: In addition to hypersensitivity to garlic, it is contraindicated for people with stomach problems and gastric ulcers. Inconvenient for newborns and nursing mothers, as well as people with dermatitis.

Warning: The use of the drug should be restricted to preparations obtained recently, without heating and preferably stored at acidic pH.

SWAMP MASTIC

Scientific name: *Schinus terebinthifolius* Raddi

Family: *Anacardiaceae*

Popular names: Aroeira, aroeira do brejo, aroeira negra, aroeira pimenteira, aroeira vermelha.

Chemical composition: The stem bark is rich in tannins, which give this plant its astringent, disinfectant and anti-inflammatory properties. It also contains resin (terembetin), terpene hydrocarbons, gallic acid and essential oils (camphene, limolene, felandrene, etc.).

Tests carried out with preparations based on stable Carbopol gels, using aqueous extracts at 1.5% and Carbopol 941, showed inhibition halos in the order of 10 mm and 20 mm in 3 standard strains of *Staphylococcus aureus: S. aureus* ATCC 6538 P, *S. aureus* ATCC 6538 and *S. aureus* ATCC 9144 .[3]

Its therapeutic action in chronic cervicitis and cervico-vaginitis has also been proven, using intravaginal tampons impregnated with aroeira hydroalcoholic extract and kept in contact with the cervix for 24 hours. It is active against Monilia and Pseudomonas.

Indications: Anti-inflammatory, healing, antimicrobial.

Part(s) used: Bark.

Directions for use: 2% decoction. Take 50 to 200 ml a day. Tincture: take 30 drops,

3 times a day. Syrup: take 3 tablespoons, 3 times a day. Ingestion of the fruit can cause poisoning with vomiting and diarrhea. Ingesting just two fruits of this plant causes inflammation of the mucous membranes and stomach irritation.

Adverse and/or toxic effects: The resin produced by this plant, in contact with the skin, causes dermatitis.

Contraindications: Pregnant women and people with a history of hypersensitivity to the plant.

BARBATENON

Scientific name: *Pithecellobium avaremotemo* Mart

Family: *Leguminaceae/Mimosoideae*

Popular names: Barbatenon, barbatim, ibatimó, bark of youth, squeezing tree.

Chemical composition:

Tannins: Around 50% in the dried bark. There are around 22 tannin compounds isolated so far.

Other: It also contains resins, mucilage and coloring substances.

Tannins are responsible for its antimicrobial, anti-inflammatory and healing activity. In tests to assess its antimicrobial activity, the extract showed a halo of inhibition in the following order: *Staphylococus aureus* (18 mm), *Pseudomonas aeruginosa* (13 mm). The extract proved to be active against *Biomphalaria glabrata* (schistosomiasis). Another study using ointment made with barbatim extract showed the same efficacy as Nebacetim.

This plant is exclusive to South America. There are 26 species, 25 of which are found in Brazil. Some of the other species of barbatenon are used for the same therapeutic purpose.

Indications: Antibacterial, anti-inflammatory, healing, anti-hemorrhagic. **Part(s) used:** Stem bark. .

How to use: For external use, you can make a decoction of the bark. For internal use, use the 20% tincture, 30 drops, three times a day or the 2% decoction, half a cup, three times a day.

Adverse and/or toxic effects: Its pods are toxic due to their high saponin content. Preparations of the bark used orally, in large quantities, cause the inactivation of digestive enzymes, making digestion difficult. Tannins, in large quantities, cause erosion of the digestive mucous membranes. In rats, the use of the seeds caused an embryotoxic effect and a decrease in the liver's energy metabolism.

Contraindications: Pregnancy and lactation

CAJUEIRO ROXO

Scientific name: *Anacardium occidentale* L.

Family: *Anacardiaceae*

Popular names: Caju, acajù, acajuiba and caju manso.

Chemical composition: Tannins and polyphenols, phenolic acids (anacardiol and anacardic acid), flavonoids (quercitin, apigenin and campeferol), essential oils such as limonene, vitamin C, etc. It has inhibitory activity against *Staphylococcus aureus, Micrococcus luteus, Proteus vulgaris, Salmonella typhi, Helicobacter pyloris, Pseudomas aeruginosa, Bacillus cereus* and *Candida albicans,* among others.

Pharmacological tests on chestnut liquid have shown that it acts against *Streptococus mutans* (tooth decay) and *Proprionibacterium acnes* (acne) **Indications**: Antibacterial, anti-inflammatory, healing, hypoglycemic, anti-bleeding.

Part(s) used: Stem bark, leaves and fruit.

How to use: For internal use, use the 2% decoction. Consume 50 to 200 ml a day. For external use, 5% decoction.

Adverse and/or toxic effects: The use of bark tea in large quantities can cause stomach pains. The nut oil (rich in cardol) causes burning and blistering of the skin. The flowers and protein particles in the fruit can cause asthma-like allergies.

Contraindications: Pregnant women and people with a history of hypersensitivity to the plant.

CIDER HERB

Scientific name: *Lippia alba* (Mill) N.E.Br.

Family: *Verbenaceae*

Popular names: Erva cidreira, falsa melissa, carmelitana, erva cidreira do campo, erva cidreira brava, salva do Brasil, salva-limâo.

Chemical composition:

Essential oil (0.5 to 1.5): Beta caryophyllene (24%), geranial (12%), neral (9%), myrcene, limolene, carvacrol and others.

Others: alkaloids, iridoids and flavonoids.

The extract has shown great efficacy against bacteria that cause respiratory infections (*Staphylococcus aureus*, *S. pneumoniae* and *S. pyogenes*), inhibiting their growth in the agar-diffusion test. It also has inhibitory activity against *Candida albicans*.

Indications: Antibacterial, digestive, calming, antispasmodic and carminative.

Part(s) used: Leaves

How to use: For internal use, use the 5% infusion, 3 cups a day, after meals. For external use, use the 10% oily solution for massages or the 5% infusion for washing the infected area.

Adverse and/or toxic effects: At the recommended doses, there are no reports of these effects in the literature.

Contraindications: At the recommended doses, there are no contraindications mentioned in the literature consulted. As a precaution, do not use too much in the first months of pregnancy.

LARGE leaf cutter

Scientific name: *Plectrantus amboinicus* (Lour) Spreng.

Family: *Lamiaceae*

Folk names: Big-leaf mint, big-leaf mint, mallow of the kingdom, scented mallow, malvarisk and malvariço.

Chemical composition:

Essential oil: Thymol, carvacrol, camphor.

Flavonoids: (quercitin and luteolin).

Other: Mucilages, aromatic acids.

The thymol and carvacrol present in the plant's essential oil have antibacterial activity, especially against microorganisms that cause respiratory tract diseases. Carvacrol has recognized germicidal, antiseptic and antifungal activity.

Indications: Antibacterial, anti-inflammatory, expectorant.

Part(s) used: Leaves.

How to use: For external use, use a 5% infusion of the leaves. Internally, use one tablespoon of the syrup, three times a day.

Adverse and/or toxic effects: At the recommended doses, there are no reports of these effects in the literature.

Contraindications: At the recommended doses, there are no contraindications mentioned in the literature consulted. As a precaution, do not use too much during the first months of pregnancy.

PURPLE IPE

Scientific name: *Tabebuia avellanedae* Lor. Ex Griseb

Family: *Bignoniaceae*

Popular names: Ipê roxo, ipê, pau d'arco, ipê preto, piùva and lapacho.

Chemical composition:

Naphthoquinones: Lapacho, alpha and beta lapachone, dehydrolapachone and others. **Anthraquinones**: 2- methyl anth**raquinone**, 2- hydroxymethyl anthraquinone and others. **Others**: Essential oils, tannins, saponins.

Lapachol shows *in vitro* activity against *Staphylococus aurus, Streptococus sp and Brucella sp.* Lapachones show activity against *Bacillus subtilis and Salmonella typhimurium.*

The naphthoquinones from Ipê roxo have bactericidal and bacteriostatic activity, due to their ability to intoxicate mitochondrial respiration and interfere with electron transport, a mechanism which is also responsible for their antitumor activity. They show activity against the penetration of *Schistosoma mansonii* larvae and molluscicidal and cercaricidal activity against *Biomphalaria glabrata and Artemia salina.*

Studies have shown that lapachol and alpha and beta lapachones are more active against candidiasis than ketoconazole. It also has antiviral activity against various *influenza* viruses.

Lapachol has been shown to be active against polio, stomatitis and herpes simplex viruses (type I and II), by interfering with the enzymatic mechanisms necessary for their replication. *In vitro*, beta lapachone has shown reverse transcriptase inhibitory activity against retroviruses related to avian miloblastosis, murine leukemia and AIDS.

In a clinical study using lapachol drops in patients aged between 21 and 45 with acute and chronic sinusitis, who had already taken antibacterial, antiphlogistic and decongestant drugs orally and, in some cases, corticosteroids directly into the sinuses, lapachol was administered through the nostrils at a dose of 3 drops in each nostril, 3 times a day, for a period of 10 to 15 days. The patients showed satisfactory clinical responses with eradication of sinusitis in 92% of cases.

Indications: Antimicrobial, anti-inflammatory, healing, immunostimulant. **Part(s) used:** The bark of the stem and the heartwood.

How to use: Take 30 drops of tincture, 3 times a day, diluted in water. For local use (gargle and mouthwash), dilute with a little water before use.

Adverse and/or toxic effects: Lapachol, in contact with the skin, can cause allergic dermatosis. Animals given high doses of lapachol have shown anorexia, weight loss, diarrhea and drowsiness. In humans, high doses cause nausea, anemia and increased prothrombin time.

In pregnant rats, at a dose of 100 mg/Kg, there was a potent abortive action as well as a teratogenic effect.

Contraindications: Pregnant women, patients taking anticoagulants and in cases of hypersensitivity.

JUAZEIRO

Scientific name: *Zizyphus joazeiro* Mart

Family: *Rhamnaceae*

Popular name(s): Juà, joà, joazeiro, laranja de vaqueiro, enjoà.

Chemical composition:

Saponins: Jujubogenin and arabinofuranosyl.

Others: Alkaloids (amphibin-D), glyceryl stearate, betulinic acid, lupeol and resins.

In in vitro experiments with plaque-forming strains *of Streptococcus mutans*, it was found that the aqueous extract of the bark of *Z. joazeiro*, at concentrations between 0.1 and 1%, destabilizes dental plaque, as well as exerting antimicrobial activity on plaque-forming bacteria. Comparison of the aqueous suspension obtained from the bark of *Z. joazeiro* at 1% with a conventional toothpaste showed greater efficiency in reducing dental plaque with the preparation from the plant. The fruit is rich in vitamin C.

Indications: Prevention of tooth decay, treatment of dandruff, skin wounds and as an expectorant.

Part(s) used: Stem bark (zest) and leaves.

How to use: To prevent tooth decay, dry the bark, pulverize it, dip a wet toothbrush in the powder and brush your teeth.

To treat dandruff and skin wounds, the affected area is washed with the bark foam. The syrup or decoction is used to treat coughs.

Adverse and/or toxic effects: Prolonged use may pose risks to the user's health due to the hemolytic action of saponins. In high doses, it produces vomiting, colic and severe irritation of the gastrointestinal tract.

It should not be used for long periods because of its strong abrasive action, which can remove tooth enamel.

Contraindications: In adequate doses and with a non-prolonged duration of use, there are no contraindications mentioned in the literature consulted.

JUCA

Scientific name: *Caesalpinia ferrea* Mart

Family: *Caesalpineacea*

Popular name(s): Jucà, jucaina, ibira-obi, muirà-obi, muiré-ita, pau-ferro- verdadeiro.

Chemical composition:

Tannins: Gallic acid, ellagic acid and methyl gallate.

Others: Betta-systosterol, alkaloids, flavonoids and essential oils.

Experimental studies with the 50% ethanolic solution of the seeds showed specific antiseptic action for *Staphylococcus aureus, Staphylococcus epidermidis* and *Escherichia coli.*

The hydroalcoholic extract of this plant showed inhibitory activity against the larval embryogenesis of the genus *Ancyslotoma.* The use of jucà bark in chronic gastric ulcers induced by acetic acid led to a reduction in the number of lesions and a reduction in the secretion of hydrochloric acid. Studies have shown the anti-inflammatory activity of the bark and fruit.

In popular circles, there are many therapeutic indications for this plant. However, there are still few pharmacological studies on it.

Indications: Antimicrobial, anti-inflammatory, healing and hypoglycemic.

Part(s) used: Bark and pods with seeds.

How to use: For external use, you can make a 5% decoction of the bark and pods. For internal use, use the 20% tincture, 30 drops, three times a day.

Adverse and/or toxic effects: The use of high doses can cause digestive symptoms such as stomach pain, diarrhea, intestinal cramps due to the high concentration of tannins.

Contraindications: Pregnant and breastfeeding women.

MORINGA

Scientific name: *Moringa oleifera Lam*

Family: *Moringaceae*

Popular names: Moringa, lirio, cedar and quina okra.

Chemical composition: The seeds of this plant contain 30% fixed oil, rich in oleic acid, which are complex polysaccharides with strong binding properties. It also contains the chemical constituents pterigospermine and rhamnosyl-oxybenzyl-isothiocyanate, which have antimicrobial effects on *Bacillus subtilis, Mycobacterium phei, Serratia maarcenses, Escherichia coli, Pseudomonas aeruginosas, Shigela and Streptococus.* For this reason, the crushed seeds are used in water treatment for their ability to agglutinate and sediment suspended particles and for their antimicrobial action.

Its leaves are rich in protein and vitamins A and C. In some regions, the leaves of this plant are used in school meals. It can also be used as animal feed.

Indications: Antibacterial, anti-inflammatory, healing.

Part(s) used: Seeds, leaves and roots.

How to use: To purify water, the seeds are bruised and placed in the container with the water. The ointment is used to treat infected wounds.

Adverse and/or toxic effects: At the recommended doses, there are no reports of these effects in the literature.

Contraindications: At the recommended doses, there are no contraindications mentioned in the literature consulted.

ROMANCE

Scientific name: *Punica granatum* L.

Family: *Punicaceae*

Popular names: Pomegranate, garnet, pomegranate, pomegranate tree.

Chemical composition:

Tannins (around 20 in the stem bark, fruit and roots): Punicalin, pulicalagin, punicofolin and others.

Alkaloids: Peletierin, methylpeletierin, pseudopeletieria and others.

Studies with aqueous and ethanolic extracts of the fruit and stem bark have shown activity against various microorganisms*: Staphylococcus aureus, Streptococus viridans, Streptococus pyogens, Bacillus anthraci, Bacillus cereus, Bacillussubtilis, Erwinia carotovora, Mycobacterium smegmatis,*

Mycobacterium phlei, Mycobacterium tuberculosis, Candida tropicalis, Candida albicans), *Cryptococcus neoformans* and *Nocardia asteroides*. With regard to its antiviral activity, *in vitro* tests have shown that the tannins in the pericarp inhibit the replication of the HSV-2 virus, which causes genital herpes.

Indications: Antibacterial, anti-inflammatory, healing, vermifuge.

Part(s) used: Bark of the fruit (mainly), stem and root, and leaves.

How to use: Internally, use the tincture, 30 drops, three times a day, or the 2% decoction, three times a day. The 5% decoction is used for gargling and mouthwash for oropharyngeal infections.

Adverse and/or toxic effects: The leaves and fruit have shown a positive hemolytic test. It can also cause cramps, vomiting and diarrhea.

The alkaloid pelletierin, present in the bark of the branches and the root, acts in a similar way to conicine and nicotine on the CNS, paralyzing the motor nerves and causing death by asphyxiation (curing action). The alkaloids, especially pelletierin, can cause nausea, vomiting, diarrhea, headaches, mydriasis (which can lead to partial blindness), vertigo, paralysis of the motor nerves, muscular weakness, visual disturbances and, in extreme cases, death by asphyxiation.

Contraindications: Due to the presence of alkaloids, it is contraindicated for use in pregnant women, as it can cause uterine contractions, leading to abortion. It is also contraindicated in nursing mothers, children and patients with a history of heart disease and kidney failure.

EXIT

Scientific name: *Kalanchoe brasiliensis* Camb.

Family: *Crassulaceae*

Popular names: Coirama, coirama-brava, saiâo and coirama-branca.

Chemical composition:

Phenolic compounds: coumaric acid, caffeic acid, ferulic acid and others.

Flavonoids: Quercitin, campeferol, rutin and others.

Others: mucilage, bryophilins A, B and C.

Studies with *K. brasiliensis* extracts showed inhibition of the growth of *Staphylococcus epidermidis*, *Micrococcus luteus, Candida albicans*, and *S. Aureus*, producing inhibition halos over 10 mm in diameter. There was also good bactericidal and fungicidal activity. With *Escherichia coli*, the halo diameter was 8.0 mm. *Bacillus subtilis,* halo of 12.3 mm. *Staphylococcus aureus*, halo of 8.6 mm. *P. aeruginosa*, 13.0 mm halo and *C. albicans,* 9.6 mm halo. The aqueous extract, at a minimum inhibitory concentration of 11.35 mg/ml, showed activity against *Candida albicans*.

Indications: Antimicrobial, anti-inflammatory, antiulcerogenic, immunomodulator.

Part(s) used: Leaves.

Directions for **use**: For internal use, take one tablespoon of the syrup three times a day.

Adverse and/or toxic effects: At the recommended doses, there are no reports of these effects in the literature.

Contraindications: At the recommended doses, there are no contraindications mentioned in the literature consulted.

12 MEDICINAL PLANTS USED TO TREAT SKIN DISEASES

In dermatology, when we prescribe a herbal medicine, we have to take into account not only the aspects relating to the plants, but also those relating to the patient's skin.

It's worth remembering that many skin symptoms are symptoms of internal diseases, the causes of which must be diagnosed and treated, in which case herbal medicine can be used as an auxiliary treatment as long as it is not incompatible with conventional treatment.

Despite the growing interest and scientific research into medicinal plants, which has proven that many of our plants can be used to treat various pathologies, most of the plants used to treat skin diseases are justified in terms of popular knowledge, pending scientific proof.

PEPPER ROSEMARY

Scientific name: ***Lippia sidoides*** Cham

Family: ***Verbenaceae***

Popular names: tray rosemary, cowboy rosemary.

Chemical composition: The essential oil obtained from its leaves consists mainly of thymol (50-60%) and carvacrol. Há other constituents in smaller quantities.

Among its fixed chemical constituents, there are some substances such as flavonoids and quinones (naphthoquinones), which have bactericidal, bacteriostatic, fungicidal and molluscicidal action. It has intense activity against *Staphylococus aureus* (skin infection).

Indications: This plant, in the form of infusions and alcoholic drinks, is recommended for external use against infected wounds, scabies, impigment on the head or body, canker sores, bad smells in the armpits and feet. It has an antispasmodic action (thymol).

Part(s) used: Leaves.

Directions for use: Infusion, alcohol, liquid soap.

Adverse and/or toxic effects: At the recommended doses, there are no reports of these effects in the literature.

Contraindications: At the recommended doses, there are no contraindications mentioned in the literature consulted.

BABOSA

Scientific name: *Aloe vera L,*

Family: *Liliaceae*

Popular names: Babosa, aloe.

Chemical composition:

Aloin* (barbaloin) - Anthraquinone compound with a stomachic and laxative action when taken in small doses and purgative in higher doses. It has anti-inflammatory activity by blocking enzymes involved in inflammatory processes.

Aloeferon - Complex polysaccharide, fibroblast stimulator. Contributes to tissue healing by inhibiting products derived from the metabolism of arachidonic acid, such as thromboxane B, limiting the production of prostaglandin F2a, preventing progressive dermal ischemia, especially in burns.

Mucilage - Contained in the liquid that oozes out when the pulp of the plant is cut. As it has a powerful moisturizing activity, it is indicated in dermatoses where there is a loss of normal moisture and greasiness of the skin and mucous membranes, which are dry and flaky to varying degrees. For example: plantar and palmar hyperkeratosis, xeroderma, cheilitis, etc.

In terms of antiviral activity, it has been shown to be active against types I and II of herpes simplex and varicella zoster.

Anti-bradykinin substance - When the skin is attacked, the cell damage releases proteolytic enzymes which, from globulins, form bradykinins, which stimulate the nerve endings, causing pain. Aloe vera contains a substance capable of blocking bradykinin.

Magnesium lactate - This substance has been shown in experiments to have an antihistamine action. Hence its effect on allergic dermatoses.

Amino acids - They work as antioxidants and immunomodulators, preventing tissue damage by free radicals, especially in skin ageing processes. We must be careful with their use in patients with malignant melanoma (skin tumor) and phenylketonuria. In the former, it has been proven that phenylalanine (an essential amino acid) is capable of promoting these tumours and in the latter, due to the congenital difficulty in metabolizing this amino acid, the patient presents, among other symptoms, eczematous dermatitis and a decrease in the pigmentation of the hair and eyes.

Studies have shown its beneficial action on irradiation injuries, as well as its preventive action on dermal freezing injuries, in this case preventing tissue necrosis, blood stasis and thrombosis.

This is due to its action on the metabolism of arachidonic acid, preventing the formation of prostaglandins and thromboxanes. In these situations, it has shown superior action to methylpredinosolone.

In addition to stimulating the production of fibroblasts, *Aloe vera* stimulates microcirculation, facilitating wound healing.

Indications: Antimicrobial, anti-inflammatory, analgesic, laxative, digestive, antipruritic, insect repellent, cicatrizant.

Part used: Inside of the leaf.

How to use: Remove the bark from the leaf and spread the oozing latex on the affected area.

Adverse and/or toxic effects: Prolonged internal use can cause digestive problems: abdominal pain, bloody diarrhea, gastric bleeding, increased incidence of colon cancer; kidney problems: albuminuria, hematuria, nephritis; hypokalemia: heart rhythm disorder, muscle cramps. This electrolyte disturbance can even increase the effect of digitalis in patients with Congestive Heart Failure (CHF). Hyperaldosteronism: weakness, slow pulse and hypothermia.

Contraindications: Pregnant women (stimulation of the large intestine produces a similar reflex effect on the uterine muscle, causing miscarriage), menstruation (can cause bleeding), children and patients with liver, kidney and intestinal problems, such as: appendicitis, ulcerative colitis, diverticulitis, Crohn's disease.

Note: Although *Aloe vera* leaf extract is considered official by several Pharmacopoeias (more or less 25 countries), the FDA (Food and Drug Administration), a US government agency, only authorizes the internal use of *Aloe*, provided the product is free of anthraquinones. There are no restrictions on its external use, which is highly effective in dermatological diseases. Therefore, internal use should be done with caution and for short periods.

CAJAZEIRA

Scientific name: Spondias mombin L.

Family: Anacardiaceae.

Popular names: Cajà, acajà, cajazeira miùda, acajaiba.

Chemical composition:

Leaves and young branches contain geraniin and galloyl-geraniin, substances of the hydrolysable tannin class, esters of caffeic acid, all of which have pronounced activity against the Herpes simplex I (cold sores) and Coxsaquii B (thrush) viruses. It is indicated for repeated attacks of painful canker sores, fever blisters and genital herpes, painful inflammations of the throat and mouth (herpetic angina).

Indications: It is indicated for repeated attacks of painful canker sores, fever blisters and genital herpes, painful inflammations of the throat and mouth (herpetic angina).

Part(s) used: Leaves and bark.

How to use: Infuse the leaves and decoct the bark.

Adverse and/or toxic effects: Not mentioned in the literature consulted.

Contraindications: Not recommended for people with a history of allergic reactions to *Anacardiaceae* (mango, cashew, umbu, cajarana, etc.).

CAPIM SANTO

Scientific name: *Cymbopogon citratus* **(**DC) Stapf.

Family: *Gramineae*

Popular names: Capim santo, capim limâo, capim cheiroso.

Chemical composition:

Essential oil: Citral, myrcene, geranial, neral, camphor, cymbopogone, cymbopogonol and others.

Others: Flavonoids (luteolin, orientin), acids (acetic, caffeic, paracumatory, chlorogenic).

Myrcene (12 % of essential oil) - Has antimicrobial, antifungal and analgesic activity.

Acetic Acid - Rubefacient, antipruritic and antiseptic, when in a concentration of 1 to 10%.

Citral (65 to 72 of the essential oil) - the main active component responsible for the soothing, antispasmodic, larvicidal and insect repellent action.

As this plant has chemical constituents with a larvicidal and insecticidal action, it can be used to control *Larva migrans* (dog worms) and to combat zoodermatoses. In the first case, it is interesting to grow the plant in areas where hookworm eggs are concentrated (e.g. gardens, backyards, etc.). In the case of zoodermatosis, it is advisable to spray the infusion or macerate of the plant in areas and at times when insects are more likely to be present.

The essential oil of this plant has antibacterial activity against *Staphylococus aureus, E. coli, Salmonella typh*, and other microorganisms. In experiments carried out in the laboratory, it was also found to have antifungal activity against around 22 species of microorganisms.

Indications: Antimicrobial, insect repellent, digestive, carminative, sedative.

Part(s) used: Leaves.

How to use: Traditionally used as an infusion.

Adverse and/or toxic effects: Not mentioned in the literature. **Contraindications**: Not mentioned in the literature consulted.

THICK-LEAF hydrangea

Scientific name: Plectrantus amboinicus (Lour) spreng.

Family: Labiatae

Popular names: Thick-leaf mint, big-leaf mint, mallow of the kingdom, scented mallow, malvarisk and malvariço.

Chemical composition

Carvacrol and thymol - They have a powerful germicidal, antiseptic, antifungal and antipruritic action. Both are compounds from the phenol group, the most powerful antibacterial agents.

Camphor - It is a cooling and repellent antipruritic, as well as being rubefacient when rubbed.

Mucilage - Edemulcent when applied to mucous membranes and emollient when applied to the skin.

Flavonoids - Some are antibacterial. Among them is quercetin, which increases hair resistance and strengthens its vitality. When the supply of these compounds is insufficient, the hair becomes fragile, with hair loss and other infections.

In addition, it is an antioxidant, inhibitor of histamine and adrenaline oxidation and stimulator of platelet production.

Indications: Antimicrobial, anti-inflammatory, expectorant. Used in treatment of coughs, hoarseness and inflammation of the mouth, gums and tonsils.

Part(s) used: Leaves

How to use: For skin diseases, you can use the juice of the plant directly on the affected area, or wash it off with the infusion. This can be used internally, as can the syrup.

Adverse and/or toxic effects: At the recommended doses, there are no reports of these effects in the literature.

Contraindications: At the recommended doses, there are no contraindications mentioned in the literature consulted. As a precaution, do not use too much in the first months of pregnancy.

SÂO CAETANO MELON

Scientific name: *Momordica charantia* L

Family: *Cucurbitaceae*

Popular names: Melâo de Sâo Caetano, erva de sâo Caetano, erva de serpente, fruta de sabià, erva de Sâo Vicente.

Chemical composition: Bitter principle, called momordoprcrin; triterpenes: momordicinins I, II and III; alkaloids, organic acids, azulene, phytosteroids and others.

Azulene - Has an anti-allergic and anti-inflammatory action, possibly due to a stabilizing effect on the mast cell membrane, either directly or indirectly, by decreasing the release of histamine and promoting the release of cortisone.

Pre-clinical and some clinical trials have confirmed its analgesic, anti-inflammatory, scabicidal and hypoglycemic action, with side effects lower than those of insulin, favoring the healing processes of the skin in patients with type II diabetes.

Indications: Skin inflammations, scabies, lice, impigens and diabetes. Antimicrobial.

Part(s) used: Leaves (mainly), flowers, fruit and seeds.

How to use: Soap, infusion and alcohol.

Adverse and/or toxic effects: Ingesting large quantities of the fruit can cause vomiting, diarrhea and hypotension due to the presence of charantin and curcubitna.

Contraindications - Do not administer preparations with the fruit during pregnancy and lactation.

FOX TAIL

Scientific name: *Conyza bonariensis* (L.) Cronquist.

Family: *Compostae*

Popular names: Foxtail, butcher.

Chemical composition:

Phenolic Acids - In general, they have an anti-inflammatory and antiseptic action. Because it contains vitamin P (bioflavonoids), it increases capillary resistance and reduces vessel permeability.

Among the phenolic acids found in this plant are:

Chlorogenic Acid - Component of aromatic polymers, which has an antifungal effect.

Caffeic Acid - Has significant antiseptic activity on the pathogenic flora that attacks the skin, especially on *Stophylococus aureus*.

Neochlorogenic Acid - With proven antifungal and bacteriostatic activity *in vitro*.

Other constituents: Flavonoids (quercetrin, quercitin, apigenin), tannins, sesquiterpene lactones, essential oil rich in limonene.

Indications: Canker sores and mycoses.

Part(s) used: Leaves.

How to use: Alcohol or leaf juice.

Adverse and/or toxic effects: At the recommended doses, there are no reports of these effects in the literature.

Contraindications: At the recommended doses, there are no contraindications mentioned in the literature consulted.

EXIT

Scientific name: *Kalanchoe brasiliensis Camb*

Family: *Crassulaceae*

Popular names: Coirama, corona, white coirama, white corona.

Chemical composition:

Flavonoids - Pigments found in plants, especially flowers, called bioflavonoids when they show pharmacodynamic activity. Among their various functions are: immunomodulatory, antioxidant, antimicrobial.

Flavonoids are indicated in almost all inflammatory and allergic skin conditions due to their immunosuppressive activity, reducing the release of mediators involved in these processes and stabilizing cell membranes.

Amino acids - Among others, arginine, which is an adjunct in the healing of some dermatoses. They have an immunostimulant, anti-cancer action and stimulate the release of growth hormone, inhibiting the loss of muscle mass and thus facilitating tissue healing.

Organic acids - Among others, we have caffeic acid, which has an antiseptic, antiplatelet and analgesic action, and coumaric acid, which improves microcirculation, promoting adequate tissue oxygenation.

Briophylline - A substance with antibiotic action against various germs: *Staphylococus aureus, Pseudomonas aeruginosas, Echerichia coli and* gram positives in general.

Indications: Anti-inflammatory, healing, antimicrobial.

Part(s) used: Leaves.

How to use: For skin diseases, you can use the juice of the plant or the ointment directly on the affected area or in the form of alcohol and syrup for internal use.

Adverse and/or toxic effects: At the recommended doses, there are no reports of these effects in the literature.

Contraindications: At the recommended doses, there are no contraindications mentioned in the literature consulted.

BUTTON BROOM

Scientific name: *Borreria verticillata* (L.) GFW Mayer

Family: *Rubiaceae*

Popular names: Botanical broom, botanical broom, friar's cord, false poaia.

Chemical composition:

Alkaloids - Emetine, borrerine and borreverine, extracted mainly from the roots of this plant. Emetine, or its derivative, dehydroemetine, with or without systemic corticoids, can reduce the pain of acute *herpes zoster*. It should, however, be used with caution due to its toxic effects.

Iridoids (valeotriates) - Responsible for the bitter taste and antibiotic action on gram-positive and gram-negative bacteria. They are most concentrated in the bark of stems and roots.

Sesquiterpene compounds - Guianene, Caryophyllene and Cadinene, found mainly in the aerial parts.

Flavonic pigments - Among others, hesperidin, which has a venotonic, vasculoprotective effect, reducing venous stasis. It also has myorelaxant activity and a CNS depressant effect.

Tannins - Because of their astringent activity, tannins precipitate skin proteins, forming a film that deprives contaminating bacteria of their nutritional substrate.

Its essential oils have antibiotic properties against gram-positive and gram-negative bacteria, and clinical trials have shown their typical effectiveness in healing impetigo lesions.

Indications: Anti-inflammatory, antibacterial, healing.

Part(s) used: The whole plant, especially the bark of the stems and roots.

How to use: Used in the form of alcohol and infusions.

Adverse and/or toxic effects: In high doses, it can cause vomiting. **Contraindications**: not mentioned in the literature consulted.

13 PLANTS WITH ACTIVITY ON THE DIGESTORY APPARATUS

ABACAXI

Scientific name: *Ananas sativus*

Family: *Bromeleacea*.

Popular name: Pineapple

Chemical constituents: Its enzyme bromalein is a mixture of bromelins A and B. It has digestive activity, comparable to the action of pepsin and papain, favoring the degradation of peptides. It also acts as a platelet antiaggregant (partially inhibits the enzyme thromboxane synthetase), fibrinolytic (activates tissue plaminogen) and anti-inflammatory (inhibits the formation of bradykinin).

It contains vitamin A, B and C, fiber, phenolic compounds, etc.

Indications: Digestive, carminative, laxative, anti-inflammatory.

Part used: Fruit.

How to use: Eat the fruit pulp with your meals. Juice can be made from the macerated peel.

Adverse and/or toxic effects: The unripe fruit causes purgative effects, a burning sensation and stinging in the mouth.

Contraindications: Patients on anticoagulants.

AROEIRA DO SERTAO

Scientific name: *Myracrodruom urundeuva Fr. All.*

Family: *Anacardeaceae*

Popular name: Aroeira do sertâo

Chemical constituents: The bark is rich in tannins and other simpler phenolic compounds. It contains two dimeric chalcones, called urundeuvins A and B, which have a strong anti-inflammatory effect. The essential oil obtained from the leaves has more than 16 constituents, the most important of which are alpha-pinene, gamma-terpinene and beta-caryophyllene. They have anti-histamine and anti-bradykinin actions.

Indications: Anti-ulcer, anti-inflammatory, healing, astringent, antimicrobial activity. In popular medicine in the north-east of Brazil, the bark of the tree trunk is one of the oldest remedies and is used for a variety of conditions.

Studies carried out with the hydroalcoholic extract in pre-clinical trials showed anti-inflammatory, healing and anti-ulcer effects. A clinical evaluation of the plant for the treatment of ulcers was carried out using aroeira elixir administered daily, orally, in the morning and evening, for 30 days to 12 individuals with gastric ulcers. At the end of the treatment, six of them showed complete healing of the ulcerative process. **Part used**: Stem bark.

Directions for use: Tincture, syrup, decoction, soap.

Adverse and/or toxic effects: In high concentrations, it can cause irritation of the gastrointestinal tract. May also cause skin allergy and respiratory allergy.

Contraindications: Patients sensitive to this plant.

BABOSA

Scientific name: *Aloe vera L.*

Family: *Liliaceae*.

Popular names: Babosa, erva babosa, caraguatâ.

Chemical constituents: Plant rich in anthraquinones (15 to 30), including babolein (20%). This compound, under the action of saprophytic anaerobic intestinal bacteria, is transformed into aloe-emodin-atrone which acts on the intestinal mucosa by decreasing the absorption of electrolytes and water, increasing peristalsis and mucous secretion. Hence its laxative and purgative action. In small doses, it has an aperitif, cholagogue and stomachic action. It also heals gastric ulcers.

It also contains resins (16 to 30%) saponins, mucilage, lignin, more than 20 minerals (calcium, magnesium, potassium, phosphorus, etc.), vitamins (A, B1, B2, B6, B9, B12, choline, etc.).

Indications: Inflammations, colds, infections, etc.

Part used: Mucilaginous juice from the leaves.

Directions for use: Alcohol juice, suppositories and ointments.

Adverse and/or toxic effects: Can cause nephritis in children when used orally. Causes fluid retention and congestion of the abdominal organs.

Contraindications: Pregnancy, patients with kidney problems and inflammatory bowel diseases.

MASHED POTATO

Scientific name: *Operculina macrocarpa L. Farwe.*

Family: *Convolvulaceae.*

Popular name: Batata de purga, jalapa do Brasil, purga do sertâo.

Chemical constituents: Its laxative action is due to the presence of resin in high concentration: 120 g per kilogram of tuber. The phenolic derivatives ferulic acid, chlorogenic acid, caffeic acid and protocatechuic acid are responsible for its antimicrobial and anti-inflammatory activity.

Indications: Laxative and purgative. It is also used to treat infectious skin diseases (impetigo and boils) and rheumatism.

Part used: Tuber.

How to use: Powder, resin and tincture.

Adverse and/or toxic effects:

Contraindication: Inflammation of the intestines, due to its irritating action on the intestinal mucosa.

BOLDO

Scientific name: *Peumus boldus Molina.*

Family: *Monimiaceae.*

Popular names: Boldo do Chile, true boldo.

Chemical constituents: The alkaloids, such as boldine* (25 to 30% of the alkaloids), sparteine and isochoridine, together with its flavonoids and the glycoside boldoglucine, have a protective action on the hepatocyte membrane, reduce mitochondrial oxidative damage and stimulate bile secretion. The essential oil (up to 2%) is rich in ascaridol (45%), cineol (30%), linalool, eugenol and p-cymene. They have antimicrobial action.

Indications: Dyspepsia, biliary dyskinesia, liver disorders, gallstones and intestinal gas.

Part used: Leaves.

Directions for use: Infuse.

Adverse and/or toxic effects: High doses of its essential oil can cause kidney irritation, vomiting and diarrhea. May cause convulsions.

Contraindications: Children, nursing mothers and patients with biliary tract obstruction. Sparteine causes uterine contractions, hence its contraindications in pregnant women.

CANELA

Scientific name: *Cinnamomum zeylanicum Blume.*

Family: *Lauraceae*

Popular name: Cinnamon, true cinnamon, Ceylon cinnamon, Indian cinnamon.

Chemical constituents: Rich in essential oil (0.5 to 3.5%). The main component is cinnamic aldehyde (60 to 75%), eugenol (10%) and other minor components such as pinene, felandrene, linalool, methyl eugenol, etc. In the leaves, the main component is eugenol (80%). It contains coumarin, mucilage, resins, gums, condensed tannins and sugars. Its essential oil stimulates enzyme production, especially trypsin, hence its eupeptic and carminative properties.

It has a protective action on the gastric mucosa, in small quantities and with a low concentration of eugenol. Otherwise, it causes gastric irritation. Pre-clinical trials have demonstrated myorelaxant and anti-inflammatory activity on smooth muscle in the trachea and ileum of guinea pigs.

In low doses, it stimulates the Central Nervous System and in high doses it has a sedative action. This activity is due to the cinnamic aldehyde.

Indications: Antimicrobial, antispasmodic (intestinal colic), eupeptic, local anesthetic.

Parts used: Bark (stem and branches) and leaves.

How to use: Infusion and decoction.

Adverse and/or toxic effects: Not mentioned in the literature. **Contraindications**: Not mentioned in the literature consulted.

CAPIM SANTO

Scientific name: *Cymbopogon citratus D.C. Staf.*

Family: *Graminae.*

Popular names: Capim santo, capim limâo, cidreira.

Chemical constituents: Its leaves are rich in essential oils containing citral, camphor, eugenol, myrcene and alkaloids such as farnesol and geranial.

Indications: Antispasmodic, antiseptic, carminative, digestive and sedative. **Part used**: Leaves.

How to use: Infuse green or dried leaves.

Adverse and/or toxic effects: At recommended doses, there are no adverse effects. At high doses, it causes irritation of the mucous membranes, increased intestinal peristalsis, tachycardia and sweating.

Contraindications: Pregnant women, nursing mothers and patients with gastric or duodenal ulcers.

CASCARA SAGRADA

Scientific name: *Rhamnus purshiana D.C.*)

Family: Rhamnaceae.

Popular names: Sacred mask, sacred bark, mask.

Chemical constituents: Rich in anthraquinone and anthracene heterosides (6 to 9%) which are formed in the leaves and stored in the older bark. The main ones are cascarosides A, B, C, D and E. Of these, A and D are the most potent. They interfere with the permeability of the mucosa, leading to the passage of liquids and electrolytes into the intestinal lumen, resulting in increased peristalsis. It contains 10 to 30% AeB alloins. Contains tannins, resins, mucilage, etc. **Indications**: Laxative, cholagogue/coleretic.

Part used: bark.

How to use: Make a decoction of the bark and take it after meals. For laboratory products, follow the instructions on the package leaflet.

Adverse and/or toxic effects: When treatment is prolonged and the dose is high, the following can occur: intestinal irritability, paradoxical constipation, nephritis, destruction of intra-colonic nerve plexuses and intestinal cancer.

Contraindications: Pregnant women, nursing mothers and patients with gastric ulcers and intestinal diseases such as ulcerative colitis and Crohon's disease.

CIDER HERB

Scientific name: *Lippia alba Mill*

Family: *Verbenaceae.*

Popular names: Erva cidreira, carmelitana, falsa melissa, cidreira.

Chemical constituents: Essential oils (0.5 to 1.5%) containing citral (calming and spasmolytic activity), myrcene (analgesic activity), linalool (anticonvulsant activity, together with citral). Its flavonoids also have a sedative effect

Indications: Intestinal cramps, poor digestion, flatulence, anxiety and insomnia.

Part used: Leaves.

Directions for use: Infuse.

Adverse and/or toxic effects: At the recommended doses, there are none. **Contraindications**: Pregnancy and lactation.

SWEET HERBS

Scientific name: *Pimpinella anisum L.*

Family: Umbelifera or Apiaceae.

Popular names: Erva doce, anis, pimpinela.

Chemical constituents: Essential oil (2 to 5%). In this, anethole (75 to 90%), estragol (methyl - chevicol), pinenolimolene, etc. Flavonoids (quercitin and apigenin) and coumarins. The pharmacological action of fennel is mainly due to anethole. It competes with dopamine, which is a prolactin inhibitor. This increases milk production. It promotes salivary and gastric secretion.

Indications: stomachic, antispasmodic, carminative, sedative and galactagogue.

Part used: Ripe seeds.

Directions for use: Infuse.

Adverse and/or toxic effects: At the recommended doses, there are no adverse and/or toxic effects.

Contraindications: Pregnant women should not take it in high doses as it can cause uterine contractions.

HOLY THORN

Scientific name: *Maytenus ilicifolia.*

Family: *Celastraceae.*

Popular names: Espinheira santa, erva santa, cancerosa, sombra de touro.

Chemical constituents:

Alkaloids: maitansine, maitanprine, maitambutine.

Flavonoids: derivatives of quercitin and campferol.

Hydrolyzable tannins*, chlorogenic acid, terpenes (maitenin, **friedelin and friedelan-3-ol**), etc. In pre-clinical studies on rats with gastric ulcers induced by indomethacin and physical stress, it showed activity against gastric ulcers comparable to ranitidine and cimetidine. It increases the volume and Ph of gastric juice. The proposed mechanism of action is inhibition of the proton pump, a common final step in the regulatory pathways of gastric secretion.

Indications: Gastritis, dyspepsia and gastric ulcers. It also has healing and antimicrobial activity.

Part used: Leaves and branches.

How to use: Infusion, tincture, alcohol, etc. There are several other forms of presentation on the market.

Adverse and/or toxic effects: Not mentioned in the literature consulted.

Contraindications: Pregnant and breastfeeding women (there are unconfirmed reports that it reduces milk production).

Note: Plant included in RENAME.

GOIABEIRA

Scientific name: *Psidium guajava L.*

Family: *Myrtaceae.*

Popular names: Guava tree, guava.

Chemical constituents: In the leaves, the main chemical constituents are tannins (9 to 10%), such as penduculagins and guacins.) There are also flavonoids (quercetin, avicularin and guajaverin) and essential oils. Effective against various microorganisms due to the tannins and flavonoids mentioned above. The bark is rich in tannins (12 to 30%).

Quercitin is mainly responsible for its anti-diarrheal activity by decreasing the production of acetylcholine, which stimulates the contraction of intestinal smooth muscles and other smooth muscles that contract involuntarily. Quercitin is most present in the bark and leaves.

Indications: Antidiarrheal, antimicrobial, hypoglycemic.

Part used: Foliar buds (eyes).

How to use: Infuse green leaf buds or bark.

Adverse and/or toxic effects: Boiling the aerial parts of this plant can show high concentrations of quercetin (44%). When the dosage reaches 800mg/Kg, mutagenic action results.

Contraindications: Pregnant and breastfeeding women.

HORTELÂ MAN

Scientific name: *Plectranthus barbatus Andr.*

Family: *Labiatae.*

Popular names: Malva santa, sete dores, boldo nacional, sete dores.

Chemical constituents: It has essential oil rich in guaiene and fenchone, bitter principles and other fixed constituents of a terpenic nature, such as barbatusin. Stimulates gastric emptying and reduces the production of HCL. Proven anti-ulcer action in rats.

Indications: Gastric ulcer, dyspepsia, stomach pain, heartburn. Stimulates appetite and digestion.

Part used: Leaves.

How to use: Infusion, alcohol, syrup or *fresh* leaf.

Adverse and/or toxic effects: In the literature consulted, there is no mention of these effects.

Contraindications: In the literature consulted, no contraindications were mentioned.

JURUBEBA

Scientific name: *Solanum paniculatum L.*

Popular Name: Jurubeba

Family: *Solanaceae*

Chemical constituents: It contains alkaloids (solanine, solanidine, solanosodine) in the roots, bark and leaves. Saponins (jurubin, paniculogenin), mainly in the roots. Solanidine and solanosodine have shown hepatoprotective activity in laboratory animals. It has a proven anti-ulcer action in pre-clinical studies by decreasing gastric secretion.

Indications: Useful in the treatment of gastric ulcers, liver and biliary tract disorders, dyspepsia, anemia and asthenia.

Parts used: Roots, stem bark, leaves and fruit.

Directions for use: Tincture, alcohol, syrup, juice, decoction and infusion.

Adverse and/or toxic effects: Internal use of the unripe fruits, or high doses of preparations of this plant, due to the presence of solanine, can cause nausea, vomiting, diarrhea, stomach aches and headaches. Avoid prolonged use.

Contraindications: Pregnant women, due to the tonic effect on the uterus.

MACELA

Scientific name: *Egletes viscosa Cass.*

Popular names: Marcela or macela-da-terra

Family: *Compositae* s.

Chemical constituents: Active ingredients: centipedic acid and ternatine (antispasmodic action) and trans-pinocarveyl acetate.

Indications: Intestinal cramps, diarrhea, dyspepsia, heartburn and migraine.

Part used: Flowers.

Directions for use: Infuse 1 to 3 % of dried flowers. Take three times a day. **Adverse and/or toxic effects**: No mention in the literature consulted. **Contraindications**: In the literature consulted, there is no reference.

MAMOE

Scientific name: *Carica papaya L.*

Family: *Caricaceae*.

Popular name: Mamoeiro

Chemical constituents: Papain, known as vegetable pepsin, a proteolytic yeast, responsible for the digestive action, can "digest" proteins up to 35 times its own weight. This substance tenderizes meat.

Chymopapain and papaya proteinase have the same function. The alkaloid carpain has an inhibitory effect on various microorganisms and on amoebae. The resins and fibers are responsible for the laxative action.

This fruit has long been used to treat people who have difficulty digesting proteins. It is also added to creams against bites and itching. The ripe fruit can be eaten raw, but the green fruit needs to be cooked.

Indications: Digestive, laxative, anti-inflammatory and vermifuge.

Part used: Fruit, milk of the green fruit, leaves and seeds.

How to use: As a laxative, eat the pulp of the ripe fruit with your meals.

Adverse and/or toxic effects: the use of large quantities of leaves can cause heart problems due to the presence of carpain. Excessive consumption of the fruit turns the hands yellow. The seeds are abortifacient and the latex of the leaves and unripe fruit irritates the skin and mucous membranes. In sensitive people, papaya produces allergic respiratory reactions.

Contraindications: In the recommended doses there are no contraindications, especially the use of the fruit.

PITANGA

Scientific name: *Eugenia uniflora*

Popular Name: Pitanga.

Family: Mirtaceae.

Chemical constituents: The leaves contain essential oils such as eugenol and cineol and phenolic acids. It also contains flavonoids (quercitin and quercitrin) and tannins.

Pre-clinical studies have shown it to have antimicrobial, mainly gram(+), antitoxidant, diuretic and antihypertensive effects. However, its most important use is in the treatment of dysentery. It increases water absorption and decreases peristaltic movements. The eugenol in the essential oil has carminative, eupeptic and antiseptic properties.

Indications: Dysentery, hypertension.

Part used: Leaves

How to use: Infuse the leaves.

Adverse and/or toxic effects: There are no known adverse effects of using Pitanga.

Contraindications: Use during pregnancy and breastfeeding is not recommended.

EXIT

Scientific name: *Kalanchoe brasiliensis Camp.*

Family: *Crassulaceae.*

Popular names: Coirama, coirama-brava, coirama branca.

Chemical constituents: Briophylline; caffeic, ferulic and cinnamic acids; steoids and flavonoids (quercitin and kaempferol). It has a high mucilage content. Laboratory studies have confirmed its anti-inflammatory, analgesic and bactericidal action.

Indications: Gastritis, ulcers, inflammations and infections.

Part used: Leaves

Directions for use: Fresh leaf juice, infusion, alcohol and syrup.

Adverse and/or toxic effects: Decrease in blood pressure.

Contraindications: Pregnant women, hypotensive patients and those with altered thyroid function.

SENA

Scientific name: *Senna alexandrina.*

Family: *Leguminosae-Caesalpinoideae.*

Popular names: Sena or sene.

Chemical constituents: Plant rich in anthraquinones, such as diatrone glycosides, senosides A and B, which are used in various laxative medicines, and aloe-emodin. It also contains flavonoids, mucilage and resins.

Indications: Laxative and antimicrobial.

Parts used: Leaves (folioli) and fruit (pods).

Directions for use: Infusion. When using laboratory medicines, follow the instructions on the package leaflet.

Adverse and/or toxic effects: When treatment is prolonged and the dose is high, the following can occur: intestinal irritability, paradoxical constipation, nephritis, destruction of intra-colonic nerve plexuses and intestinal cancer.

Contraindications: Pregnant women, nursing mothers and patients with gastric ulcers and intestinal diseases such as ulcerative colitis and Crohon's disease.

TAMARINDO

Scientific name: *Tamarindus indica L.*

Family: *Leguminosae*

Popular name: Tamarind

Chemical constituents: The flesh of the ripe fruit contains organic acids (13-15%), such as tartaric* (8-18%), acetic*, malic* and citric* acids. The leaves and roots have a high concentration of flavonoids and the seeds contain essential oils, the main ones being linoleic (55%) and oleic (15%) acids. The pulp contains a lot of sugar and pectin.

Pre-clinical studies have shown laxative activity, as well as antimicrobial activity against various germs, such as *Eschericha coli*. This is why this plant is widely used to treat urinary tract infections.

Indications: Laxative, diuretic and antimicrobial.

Parts used: Pulp of the fruit, leaves.

How to use: Juice the pulp. The leaves are infused.

Adverse and/or toxic effects: At the recommended doses, no reference in the literature consulted.

Contraindications: In the recommended doses, no reference in the literature consulted.

14 PLANTS WITH ACTIVITY IN INTESTINAL PARASITES GARLIC

Scientific name: *Allium sativum L.*

Popular names: Wild garlic, common garlic, leek.

Chemical constituents: Its main chemical constituents are allicin, alliin and ajoene. The sulphur compounds are great repellents of intestinal parasites such as *Taenia saginatta, Oxyurus, Giardia lamblia and Etamoeba histolyca.*

Indications: Vermifuge, antiseptic, antiviral.

Part used: Bulb

How to use: Garlic should be consumed raw, in the form of a 50% tincture or as a syrup. It should not be used in tea form, as high temperatures inactivate its active ingredients.

Adverse and/or toxic effects: Allicin is reasonably toxic and an irritant to the stomach. It is responsible for the characteristic smell of garlic. In high doses, it can cause headaches, burning in the gastrointestinal tract, nausea, vomiting, diarrhea, kidney problems and dizziness.

Contraindications: In addition to hypersensitivity to garlic, it is contraindicated for people with stomach problems and gastric ulcers. Inconvenient for newborns and nursing mothers, as well as people with dermatitis.

BABOSA

Scientific name: *Aloe vera.*

Popular name: Babosa.

Part used: Gel from the inside of the leaf.

Chemical constituents: Aloin or barbolein, aloe-emodin, anthran, chrysophan, etc.

Indications: Treatment for pinworms

How to use: Peel the bark off the leaf and cut into pencil-thick slices the size of two fingers. Place in the freezer and apply at night, when the worms go down into the anus. Use for a week.

Adverse and/or toxic effects: Aloe vera should not be used internally as its anthraquinone chemical constituents are toxic to the kidneys.

Contraindications: Pregnant women, nursing mothers, children and people with kidney problems.

SMALL-LEAF hydrangea

Scientific name: *Mentha x vilosa*

Family: *Labiatae.*

Popular names: Small-leaf mint, creeping mint, pot mint. **Chemical constituents**: Its main active **ingredient** is piperidone oxide, present in its essential oil in a proportion of 30 to 90 %. Other active ingredients: betacubene, limonene, 1-8 cineol, linalool, etc. Clinical trials have shown a 95% cure rate for amoebiasis, 70% for giardiasis and a high cure rate for urogenital trichomoniasis.

Indications: Antiparasitic, antiseptic, carminative, sedative.

Part used: Leaves.

Directions for use: For amoeba and giardia: one tablespoon of the syrup three times a day, or one teaspoon of the juice, on an empty stomach, for seven days.

For bad breath: Gargle with the infusion three times a day.

Adverse and/or toxic effects: No mention in the literature consulted. **Contraindications**: Not mentioned in the literature.

PEPPERMINT

Scientific name: *Mentha piperita*

Popular names: Peppermint, peppermint, mint.

Chemical constituents: Rich in essential oils (0.5 to 4%). These include menthol (33 to 55%), menthone (9 to 31%) and methyl acetate (10 to 20%). Flavonoids (12%): apigenol, rutin, hesperidin. Tannins (6 to 12%) and bitter substances.

Indications: Aperitif and eupeptic. The essential oils and flavonoids have a cholagogue, choleretic and carminative action. Useful in the treatment of amoebiasis.

Part used: Leaves.

How to use: Tea by infusion of the leaves and flowering tops, alcohol and syrup.

Adverse and/or toxic effects: Menthol can cause dyspnea, asphyxia, insomnia and nervous irritability.

Contraindications: Children, pregnant and breastfeeding women.

IPECACUANHA

Scientific name: *Cephaelis ipecacuanha Rich*

Popular names: Ipecacuanha, ipeca, papaconha, ipekaaguene (vine that makes you vomit).

Chemical constituents: Its main active ingredient is the alkaloid emetine. Other alkaloids are caffeine, ipecinine and emetamine. It also contains saponins, flavonoids and resins.

Indications: Amebicidal activity. It is probably the oldest known antibiotic active against protozoa. It is used to treat amoebic dysentery, liver abscesses caused by amoebas, coughs, bronchitis and vomiting in cases of recent ingestion of toxic substances.

Part used: Roots

How to use: Tea by decoction, tincture or syrup.

Adverse and/or toxic effects: High doses cause nausea, vomiting, cardiac and renal toxicity.

Contraindications: Pregnant women, nursing mothers, people with heart disease, neuromuscular disorders and kidney failure.

JERIMUM, PUMPKIN

Scientific name: *Curcubita maxima*

Popular name: Jerimum

Part used: Seeds

Chemical constituents: The amino acid curcubitin acts against tapeworms and inhibits the growth of young Schistosoma worms. It contains resins, vitamins A, C, B1 and B2, proteins and minerals such as calcium, iron, phosphorus, etc.

Indications: The seeds are used to treat *Ascaris lumbrichoides.* It has laxative activity (pulp). The juice of the bruised leaves is used against burns.

How to use: In popular parlance, the seeds are roasted and pounded with rapadura to form a paçoca. Take a little of this paçoca for 15 days on an empty stomach.

Adverse and/or toxic effects: Not mentioned in the literature consulted.

Contraindications: Not mentioned in the literature consulted.

MAMOE

Scientific name: *Carica papaya*

Popular names: papaya tree, papaya, pinograçu

Chemical constituents: papain, pitoquinosa, malic acid, papaiol, etc.

Part used: Seeds and fruit.

Indications: the essential oil from the seeds of the ripe fruit, which contains papayol, has a vermifuge action, especially on pinworms. For worms, use the milk of the green fruit and the seeds. An infusion is made from the green leaves.

The black, spicy seeds, which are located in the hollow, central part of the fruit, can be used as a pepper substitute. However, they can have adverse effects on the digestive system.

How to use: The seeds can be eaten *fresh.* The milk of the fruit or stem can be taken with milk or water, thirty drops on an empty stomach. In popular circles, it is common to use the milk of the fruit or stem with cachaça. The green fruit needs to be cooked. When ripe, it can be eaten *fresh.* **Adverse and/or toxic effects**: the use of large quantities of leaves can cause heart problems due to the presence of carpain. Excessive consumption of the fruit turns the hands yellow. The seeds are abortifacient and the latex of the leaves and unripe fruit irritates the skin and mucous membranes. In sensitive people, papaya produces allergic respiratory reactions.

Contraindications: In the recommended doses there are no contraindications, especially the use of the fruit.

MASTRUCTURE

Scientific name: *Chenopodium ambrosioides*

Popular names: Mastruço, mastruz, erva de Santa Maria

Chemical constituents: The seeds are rich in an essential oil, known as "kenopodium oil", which contains a volatile peroxide, ascaridol (42 to 90%) which is the active ingredient responsible for the anti-helminthic action. Chenopodium oil was widely used until the synthetic production of more effective and less toxic dewormers. Other essential oils: myrcene, felandrene, limolene. Other chemical constituents: saponins, flavonoids, vitamins B2 and C, calcium, iron and magnesium salts.

Indications: In addition to its anti-helminthic activity, especially against ascaris and hookworm, it has numerous other activities: digestive, carminative, healing, stimulating, anti-hemorrhoidal, expectorant sedative.

Indications: Vermifuge, expectorant, bone fracture healer.

Part used: Leaves and seeds.

How to use: Mastruff leaves and seeds are usually used with milk in a blender, in the morning, on an empty stomach, for 7 days. You can also use the juice.

Adverse and/or toxic effects: Skin and mucous membrane irritation, vomiting, dizziness, tinnitus, headaches, CNS depression, kidney and liver damage, temporary deafness.

Contraindications: The use of mastrux is expressly forbidden for pregnant women, due to its abortifacient properties. It is also contraindicated for children, the elderly, patients with liver or kidney dysfunction, hearing problems and debilitated people in general, as well as cardiac and gastrointestinal ulcer patients. For some years now, kenopodium oil has only been used in veterinary medicine because of its very strong toxicological action.

Treatment with mastrux should only last a maximum of one week and should be suspended for 3 or 4 weeks before being resumed.

ROMĂZEIRA

Scientific name: *Punica granatum*

Popular names: Roma, grenade, pomegranate

Family: *Punicaeae*

Chemical constituents: The bark of the root, fruit and, to a lesser extent, the trunk and branches, contain various alkaloids (peletierin, iso-peletierin and methylpeletierin) which have vermifuge activity. *In vivo* and *in vitro* activity against cestodes and nematodes. These alkaloids cause paralysis of the worms' smooth muscles and motor nerve endings. Their anthelmintic activity has been observed in humans. The slow absorption of the alkaloids hinders their toxic action. In high doses, it can cause dizziness, visual alterations and vomiting. One hour after taking pomegranate, a purgative should be taken to expel the dead worms.

Indications: Diarrhea, worms.

Parts used: Bark of the fruit, stem and roots.

How to use: Tea by decoction and infusion.

Adverse and/or toxic effects:

Contraindications: Weak people, infants or pregnant women. Do not exceed recommended doses.

11 PLANTS WITH RESPIRATORY SYSTEM ACTIVITY

Medicinal plants that act on the respiratory system can do so by fighting the micro-organisms that cause infection, reducing secretion, relaxing the bronchial muscles, facilitating expectoration, fluidizing secretions, inhibiting coughing and reducing inflammation.

Various diseases of this system can be treated with plants, many with more than one activity, such as eucalyptus, which fights infection, fluidizes secretions and reduces inflammation.

GARLIC

Scientific name: *Allium sativum* L

Family: *Liliaceae*

Popular names: Wild garlic, common garlic, leek.

Chemical constituents: Salicylic acid, citral, ajoene, allicin and alliin. Pre-clinical studies have shown the preventive action of garlic in influenza to be as effective as vaccination. The same was observed in clinical trials. Prior use of garlic capsules significantly reduced flu symptoms.

Indications: Antiviral, antimycotic, hypotensive, lipid-lowering.

Part used: Bulb

Directions for use: Adults - Take 30 drops of garlic tincture diluted in half a glass of water, 3 times a day or one small clove of garlic, two or three times a day. The use of the drug should be restricted to preparations obtained recently, without heating and preferably stored at an acidic pH.

Adverse and/or toxic effects: Allicin is reasonably toxic and a gastric irritant, responsible for the characteristic smell of garlic. In high doses it causes toxic effects on the liver and inhibits the growth of albino rats.

These effects are prevented by the use of vitamin C. In high doses, it can cause headaches, stomach aches, kidney aches and even dizziness.

Contraindications: In addition to people who are hypersensitive to garlic, it is contraindicated for people with stomach problems such as ulcers and gastritis. Inconvenient for newborns and nursing mothers, as well as people with dermatitis.

CHAMBA

Scientific name: *Justicia pectoralis.*

Family: *Acanthaceae*

Popular names: Chambà, chachambà, cumaru clover and anador.

Chemical constituents: This plant contains flavonoids (swertisin and others), coumarins, dehydrocoumarin, beta sistosterol and umbelliferone.

Umbelliferone and swertisin have a spasmolytic and relaxing action on the bronchial muscles.

Indications: Expectorant, bronchodilator, anti-inflammatory, antipyretic, analgesic and CNS depressant.

Parts used: Leaves or aerial part.

How to use: One cup of the 5% infusion, three times a day, or one tablespoon of the syrup, three times a day.

Adverse and/or toxic effects: Not mentioned in the literature. **Contraindications**: Not mentioned in the literature consulted.

CUMARU

Scientific name: *Amburana cearensis (*Allemâo) A C.Sm.

Scientific synonym: *Torresea cearensis* Allemâo.

Family: *Fabaceae*

Popular names: Umburana, imburana de cheiro, cumaru do Cearà, cumbarù das caatingas and amburana.

Chemical constituents: In the bark**:** coumarin and the flavanoid isocampeferid. In the seeds: fixed oil, coumarin, hydroxycoumarin and a protein capable of inactivating trypsin and coagulation factor XII. Both the 20% hydroalcoholic extract and the coumarin obtained from the bark of this plant showed bronchodilator action in tests on guinea pig tracheal muscle. In studies carried out on isolated guinea pig trachea, a greater direct relaxing effect was observed with the crude ethanolic extract than with coumarin. The same result was found when the preparation used was rat uterus. Laboratory tests with coumarin and a flavonoid fraction (isocampferid) showed anti-inflammatory action. Derivatives of coumarin are used as oral anticoagulants and to prevent strokes.

Indications: Anti-inflammatory, antimicrobial and expectorant.

Part used: Stem bark

Directions for use: Can be used as a tincture (30 drops dissolved in water, 3 times a day) or syrup (one tablespoon, 3 times a day) **Adverse and/or toxic effects**: Many legumes contain coumarin derivatives which are toxic. When used in large doses, they paralyze the heart and depress the respiratory center.

When the bark of the cumaru is moldy, the fungus can transform the coumarin into dicumarol, which is very toxic.

Contraindications: Due to the presence of dicumarol, which prevents clotting, use should be avoided in people with a history of bleeding and concomitant use with other medications. Best not administered to people with heart problems.

GYPSY'S THORN

Scientific name: Acanthospermum hispidum DC.

Family: *Compositae*.

Popular names: Gypsy thorn, gypsy tick, ox head. **Chemical constituents:** Diterpene glycoside, acanthospermol, hexacosanol, bertulin.

Bronchodilator action scientifically proven in pre-clinical trials. Hydroalcoholic crude extract produced inhibitory effect on contractions induced by histamine in isolated guinea pig ileum, and by oxytocin and bradykinin in isolated rat uterus.

Indications: It has a bronchodilator, hypotensive and antifungal action.

Part used: Root.

Directions for use: Use one tablespoon of the syrup, 3 times a day.

Adverse and/or toxic effects: The sprouts and seeds have shown toxic effects such as diarrhea, respiratory difficulty, hair loss, hemorrhage, limb weakness and jaundice.

Contraindications: Avoid use in cardiac patients, as increased cardiac activity has been observed in laboratory animals.

EUCALYPTUS

Scientific name: *Eucaliptus globulus* Labil.

Family: *Myrtaceae.*

Popular names: Eucalyptus, fever tree, white mahogany.

Chemical constituents: Eucalyptol, taken orally or inhaled, has expectorant, fluidifying and antiseptic activity on bronchial secretions. Menthol produces a refreshing sensation on the nasal mucosa. Regardless of the route of administration, essential oils are mostly eliminated by the respiratory tract, hence their action in respiratory pathologies.

A clinical study has shown that eucalyptus increases ciliary movement in patients with chronic obstructive bronchitis. However, continued use can have an immobilizing effect. It has a febrifuge action.

Indications: Used in the treatment of sinusitis, bronchitis and other infections of the respiratory system.

Part used: Leaves

Directions for use: Infuse the leaves at 2.5%. Take one cup three times a day.
Adverse and/or toxic effects: High doses can cause: nausea, vomiting, epigastralgia, gastroenteritis, suffocation, hematuria, neurotoxicity (convulsions, loss of consciousness, delirium and miosis). In more serious cases, respiratory bulbar depression and coma. In asthmatic children, a paradoxical effect (bronchospasm) may appear. Used topically, the essential oil can cause urticaria and eczema.

Contraindications: Do not use in epileptics, pregnant women and children under 3 years of age.

GUACCO

Scientific name: *Mikania Glomerata,*

Family: *Compositae*

Popular names: Guaco, guaco cheiroso, erva de cobra, coração de Jesus.

Chemical constituents: Rich in coumarin and its derivatives. Other chemical constituents are: essential oils (beta-caryophyllene, germacrene, bicyclogermacrene) tannins, flavonoids and saponins. Coumarin relaxes the smooth muscles of the respiratory tree, which is where its spasmolytic and bronchodilating action comes from.

Pre-clinical studies *in vitro* with isolated guinea pig trachea contracted by histamine showed a relaxing effect. The same effect was obtained with human muscle, pre-contracted with K+.

Indications: Expectorant, analgesic, antitussive, anti-inflammatory and antiseptic.

Part used: Leaves.

How to use: For respiratory ailments, use the syrup. In the treatment of neuralgic and rheumatic pains, the leaves can be ground, compressed or used as an ointment.

Adverse and/or toxic effects: In the indicated doses, it does not cause them. At high doses, it causes tachycardia, vomiting and diarrhea.

Contraindications: Pregnant women and children.

Note: Plant included in RENAME

LARGE-LEAF hydrangea

Scientific name: *Plectrantus amboinicus Lour.*

Family: *Lamiaceae*

Folk names: Thick-leaf mint, large-leaf mint, Bahia mint, mallow of the kingdom, scented mallow, malvarisk and malvariço.

Chemical constituents: Essential oils (thymol and carvacrol), flavonoids and mucilages, which are responsible for its antiseptic, broncho-dilating, mucolytic and anti-flammatory activities. As a result, there is an improvement in respiratory tract pathologies. Carvacrol has a recognized germicidal, antiseptic, bronchodilating, mucolytic and antifungal action.

Indications: Antiseptic, anti-inflammatory, expectorant.

Part used: Leaves

Directions for use: Take one tablespoon of the syrup three times a day or one cup of the infusion three times a day. For mouth diseases with infection and inflammation, rinse and gargle the infusion three times a day.

Adverse and/or toxic effects: At the recommended doses, there are no references to these effects in the literature consulted.

Contraindications: No reference in the literature consulted.

PURPLE IPE

Scientific name: *Tabebuia avellanedae* Lor.

Family: *Bignoniaceae*.

Popular names: Ipê roxo, ipê, pau d'arco, ipê preto, piùva and lapacho.

Chemical constituents: Its main chemical constituents are naphthoquinones, including lapachol, alpha and beta lapachone. Other chemical constituents: B-lapachone, carobin, carobinase and tannins. There are also essential oils, antaquinones, saponins, flavonoids, bitter substances, etc. Naphthoquinones, such as lapachol, have a strong inhibitory effect on various microorganisms that cause respiratory infections. Their mechanism of action is through mitochondrial intoxication of microorganisms. In a clinical study with patients aged between 21 and 45, suffering from sinusitis in the acute and chronic phases, who had already used antibacterial, antiphlogistic and decongestant drugs orally and in some cases corticoids directly into the sinuses, lapachol was administered through the nostrils, at a dosage of 3 drops in each nostril, 3 times a day for a period of 10 to 15 days. The patients showed satisfactory clinical responses with eradication of sinusitis in 92% of cases.

Indications: Antimicrobial, anti-inflammatory, healing.

Parts used: Stem bark and heartwood

How to use: Take 30 drops of tincture, 3 times a day, diluted in water. For local use (gargling and mouthwash), use the decoction. In the treatment of sinusitis, it can also be inhaled alone or in combination with other plants, such as eucalyptus.

Adverse and/or toxic effects: Contact of the sprayed substance with the skin can cause allergic dermatosis. Tests on rats have shown both Lapachol and B-Lapachone to be toxic, including abortifacient and teratogenic effects. In high doses it can cause gastrointestinal problems, anemia and increased clotting time.

Contraindications: Pregnant women and in cases of hypersensitivity.

MASTRUZ

Scientific name: *Chenopodium ambrosioides* L.

Family: *Chenopodiaceae*

Popular names: Mastruz, mastruço, erva de Santa Maria, menstruz, lombrigueira and erva mata-pulgas.

Chemical constituents: Its chemical composition includes essential oil (rich in ascaridol), saponins, flavonoids, etc. Expectorant and fluidifying activity in lung diseases. It is a vermifuge (helminths), cholagogue, emmenagogue, abortifacient and antimicrobial.

Indications: Expectorant, vermifuge, antiseptic. Helps consolidate bone fractures.

Used parts: Leaves and seeds.

How to use: Infuse 3g in 250ml of hot water. Take 3 cups a day.

Green leaf juice: 2g in 1 cup of sweetened milk.

Adverse and/or toxic effects: Mastruz oil is very toxic to the liver and kidneys due to the presence of ascaridol. Treatment with mastruz should not be prolonged due to its toxicity.

Contraindications: Children, the elderly, the frail, pregnant women and patients with hearing disorders.

MILONA

Scientific name: *Cissampelos sypodialis.*

Family: *Menisperm.*

Popular names: Milona, jaguar ear.

Chemical constituents: Plant rich in alkaloids such as warifteine, milonine and laurifoline, the former being the most commonly found.

Pharmacological tests on rats showed relaxing effects on tracheal smooth muscle, with inhibition of spontaneous tone and contractions induced by asthma mediators. It has also been shown to act on the gastrointestinal tract (ileum), reproductive system (uterus) and vascular system (aorta).

It has a bronchodilator action and inhibits the degranulation of neutrophils in human cells induced by the peptide formyl-methionine-proline-leucine. This mechanism of action involves an increase in intracellular levels of cyclic adenosine monophosphate, resulting in the inhibition of nucleotide phosphoesterase enzymes.

Indications: Bronchodilator, expectorant, fluidifier.

Parts used: Roots and leaves.

How to use: One cup of the infusion of the leaves or the decoction of the roots, three times a day. Thirty drops of the tincture, three times a day, or a spoonful of the syrup, three times a day.

Adverse and/or toxic effects: At the recommended doses, there are no references to these effects in the literature consulted.

Contraindications: There are no references in the literature consulted.

MUSSAMBÊ

Scientific name: *Cleome spinosa* Jacq.

Family: *Caparidaceae.*

Popular names: Mussambè, Sete-marias, Mussambè-cor-de-rosa, Bredo- fedorento.

Chemical constituents: In the literature we consulted, there is no record of scientific studies on its chemical constituents and its therapeutic action, but its use is widespread in popular circles. The plant is commonly used in the form of a flower lick to reduce coughing and increase expectoration. It also has a bronchodilator effect.

Indications: Expectorant, antitussive.

Used parts: Flowers, leaves, root and seeds.

How to use: Decoct the roots and seeds and infuse the leaves and flowers at 3%. Take 1 cup, 3 times a day.

Adverse and/or toxic effects: When used in excess, the seeds cause intestinal gas.

Contraindications: There are no references in the literature consulted.

TRANSFER

Scientific name: *Plantago major L*

Family: *Plantaginaceae*

Popular names: Transagem, tanchagem.

Chemical constituents**:** Its main chemical constituents are chlorogenic and neochlorogenic acids, aucubin and mucilage.

Chlorogenic and neochlorogenic acids are responsible for the anti-inflammatory and healing action. Aucubin is responsible for the antimicrobial action on *Staphylococus aureus and Micrococus flavus.* Studies on guinea pigs have shown its bronchodilator effect on bronchial muscle spasm induced by acetylcholine.

Indications: Antiseptic and anti-inflammatory. It has hypotensive activity and reduces plasma cholesterol.

Parts used: Leaves and seeds

How to use: Gargle and rinse the infusion of its leaves to treat inflammation of the oropharynx. The infusion and syrup can be taken to treat bronchospasm.

Adverse and/or toxic effects: At the recommended doses, there are no references to these effects in the literature consulted.

Contraindications: No reference in the literature consulted.

15 PLANTS WITH ORAL HEALTH ACTIVITY WATERCRESS OF PARA

Scientific name: *Spilanthes acmella*

Family: *Asteraceae.*

Popular names: Watercress, water pepper, anesthesia, jambu.

Chemical constituents: Saponins, triterpenoids, spilanthol (responsible for the anesthetic action) and essential oils (responsible for the characteristic smell) are its main chemical constituents.

Indications: Analgesic (toothache), antiseptic, disinfectant.

Parts used: Flower buds and leaves.

How to use: Place the bruised bud or cotton wool soaked in alcohol on the area of the tooth that is sore, or on the aphtha. As an antiseptic, you can rinse your mouth with the infusion.

Adverse and/or toxic effects: In the recommended doses and form of use, there are no adverse/toxic effects reported in the literature.

Contraindications: Avoid contact with the larynx because of the risk of causing paralysis of the glottis which, although transient, can be dangerous.

PEPPER ROSEMARY

Scientific name: *Lippia sidoides Cham*

Family: *Verbanaceae.*

Popular names: Alecrim de tabuleiro, estrepa cavalo, alecrim do Nordeste. **Chemical constituents:** Contains essential oil rich in thymol (50 to 60%) and carvacrol (5 to l0%), which are responsible for the spicy taste and strong odor. The essential oil has considerable action against bacteria that cause tooth decay and other oral pathologies. In laboratory experiments, it showed a halo of inhibition comparable to that caused by antibiotics such as vancomycin and cephaloxin.

Indications: Antiseptic, bad breath, canker sores, inflammation of the gums and tonsils.

Part used: Leaves.

How to use: Mouthwash with the infusion or the tincture diluted in water, three times a day.

Adverse and/or toxic effects: No reference in the literature consulted. **Contraindications**: No reference in the literature consulted.

CALENDULA

Scientific name: *Calendula officinalis* L.

Family: *Asteraceae.*

Popular names: Calendula, marigold, garden wonder.

Chemical constituents: Its chemical composition includes essential oils, saponins, quercitin, sitosterol, salicylic acid, inulin, tannins and phenolic acid.

Pre-clinical and clinical studies have demonstrated its anti-inflammatory and antimicrobial activity, as well as increased epithelialization of wounds. It also induces micro-vascularization.

Indications: Anti-inflammatory, antimicrobial and healing.

Part used: Flowers.

How to use: Gargle with an infusion of the leaves three times a day.

Adverse and/or toxic effects:

Contraindications: Pregnant women, due to its effect of provoking uterine contractions.

CHAMOMILE

Scientific name: *Chamomilla recutita*

Family: *Asteraceae.*

Popular names: German chamomile, common chamomile.

Chemical constituents: Essential oils (0.3 to 1.5%): azulenes (26-46%), mainly camazulene and guajazulene. Other components: **bisabolol**, mucilages, tannins, coumarins, flavonoids (**apigenin**, quercitin, patuletin). **Indications:** Analgesic (in dental eruptions), anti-inflammatory (tonsillitis, gingivitis, stomatitis).

Part used: Flower capsules.

How to use: Gargle with the flower infusion three times a day. **Adverse and/or toxic effects**: In high doses, it causes nausea, vomiting and insomnia.

Contraindications: There are no contraindications mentioned in the literature consulted.

CRAWBERRY OF INDIA

Scientific name: *Eugenia caryophyllus*

Family: *Myrtaceae.*

Popular names: Clove, clove.

Chemical constituents: Essential oils (15-20%). These include eugenol (65-90%). There is also eugenyl acetate (5-20%), methylaminacetone and caryophylline.

Indications: Analgesic (toothache), anti-inflammatory, antimicrobial **Part used:** Dried flower bud.

How to use: Place the bruised bud or a cotton pad soaked in the tincture on the sore tooth area. As an antiseptic and anti-inflammatory mouthwash, the infusion should be rinsed out.

Adverse and/or toxic effects: The essential oil in high doses causes irritation of the mucous membranes and neurotoxicity.

Contraindications: Patients with gastric ulcers.

GINGER

Scientific name: *Zingiber officinale Rose.*

Family: *Zingiberaceae.*

Popular name: Ginger.

Chemical constituents: The plant contains essential oils (0.5 to 3%), the main ones being camphene (8%), alpha-pinene (2.5%), cineol and zingiberene. It has resins (5 to 8%), where the bitter and spicy principles are concentrated, which are responsible for the antispasmodic and antiemetic action.

The rhizome extract, rich in essential oils, is very active against various microorganisms, some of which are responsible for respiratory and mouth infections. It has anti-inflammatory and antipyretic activity.

Indications: Antiseptic and anti-inflammatory. Reduces hoarseness. Used in genitourinary tract infections and as an appetite and gastric secretion stimulant. It has a carminative, antiemetic and antispasmodic action.

Part used: Rhizome.

Directions for use: In cases of pharyngitis, chew small pieces.

Warning: Contact with skin can cause blisters similar to burns. Therefore, use caution.

Adverse and/or toxic effects: At the recommended doses, there are no references to these effects in the literature consulted.

Contraindications: Pregnant women, nursing mothers and patients with vesicular lithiasis.

JOAZEIRO

Scientific name: *Zizyphys joazeiro*

Family: *Rhamnaceae*.

Popular names: Joà, juà.

Chemical constituents: Saponin-rich plant with proven antiseptic action. Destroys bacterial plaque, responsible for the formation of cavities. **Indications:** Antiseptic, expectorant and mucolytic.

Part used: Zest.

How to use: Brush your teeth with the zest. To expectorate coughs, use the syrup. To treat wounds on the skin and scalp, use it as soap.

Adverse and/or toxic effects: In high doses, it can cause nausea, vomiting and intestinal cramps.

Contraindications: Pregnant women and children.

TOMATO

Scientific name: *Lycopersicon esculentum* Mill.

Family: *Solanaceae*.

Popular name: No other popular name.

Chemical constituents: Tomatidine, tomatine, solanidine, rutin, chlorogenic acid, lycopene and furocoumarin. Tomatine is antifungal, with good action against candida.

Indications: Anti-inflammatory, antifungal (candida).

Part used: Pulp.

How to use: For candidiasis, bruise the pulp and leave it in the mouth for a while.

Adverse and/or toxic effects: There are no references in the literature.

Contraindications: There are no references in the literature.

16 TOXIC PLANTS

These are all plants which, when in contact with the organism of humans or animals, cause damage that is reflected in the health and vitality of these beings. Every plant is potentially toxic.

The toxic principle consists of a chemically well-defined substance or group of substances, of the same or different nature, capable of causing intoxication when it comes into contact with the body.

Factors that determine or influence plant toxicity

a) **related to the plant**:

1- Environmental conditions: climatic conditions (temperature, humidity level, day length), soil (soil composition, PH, excess or lack of nutrients) and cultivation: periods of prolonged drought favor the accumulation of toxic substances due to the decrease in metabolism.

2- Part of the plant: in some plants, there is a higher concentration of the toxic principle in one or more parts of the plant. E.g. *Ricinus communis* (castor bean) - seeds.

3- Variety of plant: within the same species there can be variations in the concentration of toxic principles contained in a plant.

4- Solubility of the active ingredient: intoxication can be precipitated by drinking water. E.g.: *Polycourea marcgravii* (rat grass) - monofluoracetic acid.

b) **related to the person**:

1- Age: children and the elderly are more susceptible to poisoning.

2- Dose: the higher the dose, the greater the likelihood of poisoning.

3- Health conditions: weakened organisms are more susceptible to poisoning.

4- Route of administration: many plants for external use are toxic when administered orally. E.g. Comfrey (*Synphytum officinale* L.).

5- Special physiological conditions: Hypersensitivity of the user, pregnancy, etc. Many plants considered medicinal are abortifacients or can harm the fetus. E.g.: Comfrey (*Synphytum officinale* L.), Mussambê (*Cleome heptaphilla*), Holy Grass (*Cymbopogon citratus* (D.C.) Stapf).

6- Time of use: the longer the time of use, the more prone the user is to toxic problems.

Disorders caused by toxic plants:

1- Digestive disorders: nausea, vomiting, abdominal cramps, diarrhea. The main culprits for these symptoms are:

a) Toxic proteins: Ricin from castor beans (*Ricinus comunis* L).

b) Solanines: found in the genus *Solanum* (Horse-breast, Jurubeba, Moor-grass, etc.)

c) Saponins: *Sapindus saponaria* L. (Soap).

d) Resins: a mixture of alcohols, acids and phenols have an irritating effect on the gastrointestinal tract. Ex: *D. racemosa* Grisele (Imbira) causes severe diarrhea.

2 **- Cutaneous-mucosal disorders**:

Mechanical trauma: e.g. *Stipa sp* - spiky fruits pierce the skin.

Primary chemical irritation: milky sap from hazelnuts, the Crown of Christ, etc.

Allergic sensitization: Ipê roxo, aroeira do sertao.

Photosensitization: Plants rich in furocoumarins: Rue and Hypericum.

Mucosal disorders such as erosions, bleeding ulcers, edema. E.g. *Dieffenbachia picta Schott.*

3 **- Respiratory Allergies**:

Allergic rhinitis, allergic asthma. Ex: *Ricinus communis* (castor bean).

4 **- Hallucinations:** black jurema, angico, white skirt, coca, etc.

Types of poisoning

1- **Acute poisoning**: almost always due to accidental ingestion of the whole plant or parts of it. Its incidence is preponderant in the pediatric group.

2- **Chronic Poisoning**: **(three types)**

a) Continued ingestion: Continued ingestion of certain plant species causes clinical disorders, often complex and serious. For example: liver cirrhosis caused by the habit of eating Crotalària and liver and circulatory disorders caused by the habit of eating food prepared with wheat flour contaminated with Senecium seeds, observed in some oriental populations.

b) Chronic Exposure: Evidenced in particular by skin manifestations due to systematic contact with plants, seen more frequently in industrial or agricultural activities.

c) Continued use of certain plant species, in the form of inhalation powders, smokes or infusions, in order to experience hallucinogenic and narcotic effects.

Basic rules of prevention when in contact with plants.

- Get to know the dangerous plants in your area, house and yard. Know them by appearance and name.
- Do not eat wild plants, including mushrooms, unless they are well identified.
- Keep plants, seeds, fruit and bulbs away from small children.
- Teach children as early as possible not to put plants or their parts in their mouths, warning them about the potential dangers of toxic plants.
- Do not allow children to suck or chew seeds or any other part of the plant.
- Identify plants before eating their fruit.
- Don't trust animals or birds to know if a plant is toxic.
- Remember that heating or cooking does not always destroy the toxic substance.
- Store bulbs and seeds safely and away from children.
- Do not make or take home remedies with plants without medical advice.
- Remember that there are no safe tests or rules of thumb for distinguishing edible plants from poisonous ones.
- Avoid smoke from plants that are being burned unless they are clearly identified.

General principles for treating acute plant poisoning

The treatment of any acute poisoning, including plant poisoning, should follow the 4 basic stages: reducing the body's exposure to the toxicant, increasing the elimination of the toxicant already absorbed, administering antidotes and antagonists and general and symptomatic treatment.

Thus, it can be said that a plant can be either medicinal or toxic, depending on factors related to the individual and the plant.

17 POTENTIALLY TOXIC PLANTS

AVELÓS

Scientific name: ***Euphorbia tirucalli*** L.

Family: *Euphorbiaceae*

Popular name: Avelós

Symptoms of intoxication: the lesions are initially characterized by edema and erythema, evolving into the formation of vesicles and plagues, usually pruritic and painful. Cases of ingestion of the plant are rare and the symptoms of this form of intoxication appear quickly with irritation of the oral mucosa, with a burning sensation, edema, pain and salivation. Ingestion causes severe gastroenteritis with severe diarrhea and vomiting.

Treatment: Treatment is symptomatic. Hygiene measures (prolonged washing of the site), when there is contact with the skin, precautions against secondary infections, in the event of the formation of vesicles and pus. In contact with the eyes, after prolonged washing with a large amount of water, the use of antiseptic eye drops is recommended. In more serious cases, the use of corticoids and antihistamines is also recommended. In cases of ingestion, gastric lavage is only recommended if the quantity of the plant ingested is considerable. The administration of activated charcoal and laxatives is indicated, as well as analgesics and demulcents.

Toxic part: Leaf latex

MEADOWSWEET

Scientific Name: ***Dieffenbachia picta*** Schott

Family: *Araceae*

Popular name: Comigo-nuém-pode.

Symptoms of poisoning: when swallowed or chewed, it causes marked irritation of the mucous membrane of the mouth and pharynx, with swelling of the lips, tongue and gums. Burning pain and intense salivation make speaking and swallowing difficult. Sometimes there are also signs of esophagitis, with burning, as well as vomiting and abdominal cramps.

Treatment: milk or egg white can be administered at home and the patient taken immediately to the nearest hospital.

Toxic parts: The whole plant, particularly leaves and stems.

SPIRAL

Scientific name: ***Nerium oleander L***.

Family: *Apocynaceae*

Popular name: Espirradeira.

Symptoms of poisoning: begins with gastrointestinal disorders (nausea, vomiting, abdominal cramps and mucus-bloody diarrheal bowel movements) followed by cardiac and neurological disorders (drowsiness, dizziness, visual disturbances and coma).

Treatment: Requires emergency treatment. Take the patient immediately to the nearest hospital. The therapeutic approach in cardiac patients depends on the electrocardiographic tracings. Flushing should be carried out carefully. Digestive disorders should be treated symptomatically.

Toxic parts: The whole plant.

MAMONA

Scientific Name: ***Ricinus communis L***

Family: *Euphorbiaceae*

Popular names: Mamona, carrapateiro.

Symptoms of poisoning: Intense irritation of the mucous membranes, with destruction of epithelial cells, nausea, intense vomiting, abdominal cramps and bloody diarrhea. This is followed by severe hydro-electrolytic disorders, hypotensive states, shock and acute renal failure. The main toxicant is the alkaloid ricin found in the pulp of the seed.

Treatment: the most important measures are vomiting and gastric lavage.

Toxic part: Seeds.

WHITE URTIGA

Scientific name: ***Urtiga urens L.***

Family: *Urticaceae.*

Popular name: White nettle

Symptoms of poisoning: skin and mucous membrane lesions appear quickly after contact with the plant. Characteristically, the lesions are limited only to the exposed areas and are of the urticating and vesicant type, with erythemas, blisters and vesicles that are very itchy or painful.

Treatment: treatment is only symptomatic with the application of antiseptic and protective solutions, as well as the administration of oral antihistamines to relieve itching and analgesics when necessary.

Toxic parts: Hairs present on the leaves.

YUCCA BRAV A

Scientific name: *Manihot utillissima Pohl.*

Family: Euphorbiaceae

Popular name: Mandioca-brava

Chemical constituents: **Symptoms of poisoning**: start with gastrointestinal disorders such as nausea, vomiting and abdominal cramps, followed by headache, dizziness, respiratory disorders and convulsions. Seizures usually precede death.

Treatment: measures should be taken immediately. In addition to measures to induce vomiting and gastric lavage, these should be carried out with caution, especially if the patient has severe neurological disorders. Take the patient immediately to the nearest hospital.

Toxic parts: All parts. However, the toxic principle is more concentrated in the root bark and in the milky latex. The toxic principle is a glycoside, which upon hydrolysis releases cyanide acid (HCN).

WHITE SKIRT

Scientific name: *Datura Stramoniun.*

Family: *Solaneceae*

Popular names: trumpet, lady-of-the-night.

Symptoms of intoxication: mild cases of intoxication are characterized by nausea, vomiting, visual impairment and dry mouth. In more serious cases, the symptoms are as follows: blurred vision, photophobia with pupil dilation, dry mucous membranes, fever, skin hyperemia, palpitations, hallucinations, disorientation, respiratory disorders, convulsions and coma.

Treatment: if treatment is swift and successful, the acute symptoms begin to disappear within 12 to 48 hours, but the mydriatic effect (pupil dilation) persists and can last for several weeks. Emergency measures are: administration of activated charcoal, inducing vomiting and taking the patient immediately to the nearest hospital.

Toxic parts: All parts of the plant.

Note: In order to prevent plant poisoning, it is necessary to take preventive measures, such as: publicizing the most common toxic species as much as possible and through all means of communication; recommending the need for medical advice when using any plant preparation for medicinal purposes; educating the population about the inconvenience of ingesting or handling any unknown plant species; informing yourself about the toxicity of the plants in your surroundings and remembering that there are no practical rules or safe tests to distinguish edible plants from poisonous ones.

If poisoning occurs in our state, immediately call CEATOX (Toxicological Information Center), which has a permanent office located at the Lauro Wanderley University Hospital, for advice, on 3216-7007.

18 MEDICAL PRESCRIPTION OF HERBAL MEDICINES

The medical prescription of herbal medicines is made to cure or alleviate diseases or symptoms. In biomedicine, the prescription is based on a nosological diagnosis (e.g. bronchitis) or a symptomatic diagnosis (cough).

In phytotherapy, much of the knowledge about the medicinal use of plants comes from empirical observations, passed on orally over the years. As a result, most medical prescriptions for herbal medicines are made orally or with prescriptions using popular names and omitting scientific nomenclature.

Nowadays, scientific research has contributed to proving the great therapeutic potential of medicinal plants.

Once approved by the scientific community, the herbal medicine is indicated and prescribed with the same characteristics as other medicines. An example of this is the large number of herbal medicines used in orthomolecular medicine, such as *Gingko biloba.*

Medicinal plants, to a greater or lesser extent, are part of all therapeutic systems. Either by using their energetic potential, in the case of Homeopathy and Traditional Chinese Medicine; or as a complement to nutrients, such as vitamins and minerals, in the case of diet therapy; or as an antioxidant, in the case of Orthomolecular Medicine, or through their active principles as antimicrobial, anti-inflammatory, antispasmodic, etc., in Phytotherapy and Allopathy.

When prescribing herbal medicines, we must rely mainly on scientific proof of their efficacy, safety and effectiveness. This is done on the basis of pre-clinical tests, which are carried out to observe acute, sub-acute and chronic toxicity, evaluate teratogenicity and prove pharmacological action, and clinical tests, when their beneficial action and lack of toxicity are observed in humans.

In practice, most plants and phytotherapics do not fully demonstrate this, correlating pre-clinical and clinical data. Several factors, such as the diversity of medicinal plants, the lack of financial resources in the regions where they are used and the lack of interest from the pharmaceutical industry, explain this.

In the absence of scientific proof, we can use popular knowledge. Here it is important to investigate whether the indication of the plant is something old and has been maintained over time, whether it is used with this indication in many places and by many people, and whether the reports of its use corroborate its efficacy and safety.

19 THE STATUTE OF LIMITATIONS ITSELF

1 .- **Scientific nomenclature:** the genus, species and family to which the plant belongs. E.g. *Lippia alba* N.E. Brown. Family: *Verbanaceae*

2 .- **Popular name:** the popular name of the prescribed plant in the region should be clearly written next to the scientific name. Ex: *Lippia alba* N.E. Brown (lemon balm)

3 **Mode of use:** explain the route of use and dosage. Here, it is important to convert the standard measures into homemade ones. Ex: 150ml = 1 glass (American); 150ml = 1 cup (large); 50ml = 1 cup (small); 15ml = 1 tablespoon; 10ml = 1 dessert spoon; 5ml = 1 teaspoon; 2.5ml = 1 coffee spoon.

Special situations should be noted and clearly described. In the case of external use, make it clear where on the body the medicine should be applied.

3.1 - **Internal use:** for teas, juices, syrups, tinctures,

alcohol.

3.2 - **External use:** for compresses, poultices, plasters, ointments.

4 **Method of preparation: a** detailed description should be given when prescribing herbal medicines to be made at home.

5 - **Relationship with habits:** in cases where the administration of herbal medicines requires appropriate conditions that could lead to adverse reactions, clarifying instructions should be included in the prescription. For example: - Do not take a sitz bath on a full stomach, do not inhale in a ventilated area, do not apply a hot compress in a draughty environment.

20 OTHER CONSIDERATIONS

The therapist should also be aware of the following aspects:

1 .- Adverse effects

Popular belief is that, as the plant is natural, if it doesn't do any good, it won't do any harm. This is not true. Many plants are known to contain substances that are highly toxic to humans and can cause death, such as strychnine, found in the *Strychnos nux vomica* plant.

Popular knowledge, transmitted orally, needs to be scientifically proven to validate the efficacy of plants and their safety. The combination of these two types of knowledge promotes progress in the field of herbal medicine.

2 .- Interactions

Interactions between herbal medicines and synthetic or homeopathic medicines can result in the potentiation of one action or the annulment of another.

For example - plants rich in camphor act as antidotes to the action of the homeopathic medicine.

- aspirin taken with elderberry tea potentiates the antipyretic action and can cause severe hypothermia, especially in children under 1 year of age.

Plants rich in coumarin can potentiate the platelet antiaggregant activity of some allopathic drugs.

3 .- Contraindications

3.1 . Children under 1 year of age: Except for those plants known to have no toxic or adverse effects, herbal medicines should not be used in children under this age.

3.2 - Elderly: exclude plants known to be hepatotoxic, nephrotoxic and hemorrhagic (coumarins).

3.3 - Pregnant women: This group should be given special care. Tannins are abortifacients and most plants contain them. Plants with an intensely bitter taste, such as those containing quinones, are mostly abortifacients.

5. 3.4 - Other groups to consider: Nursing mothers, diabetics, people with kidney or heart failure.

21 PLANT SPECIES, GENERAL INDICATIONS

Introduction

Phytotherapy is the use of medicinal plants to prevent and treat diseases, and is the oldest and most fundamental form of medicine on Earth.

Since animals first appeared on Earth, they have instinctively used certain plants for food, healing or even to stimulate vomiting and eliminate harmful substances.

For over 6000 years, man has been instinctively testing and choosing the best medicinal plants to cure his illnesses. In the last century, medicine has spread the use of antibiotics and allopathic remedies, and our natural medicine passed down from generation to generation has been forgotten. However, every day, plants are gaining ground as allies in the physical rebalancing of the human being: the predominance of the color green is related to health and balance, the keys to a healthy man; the various shades of flowers complement this mission, bringing joy and optimism (yellow and red), peace (white), love and fraternity (pink), spirituality (violet) and harmony (blue).

Phytotherapy is a therapy that can help to cure ailments in depth and in full, in a cheap (medicine prices are "on the moon") and non-aggressive way, because it stimulates the body's natural defenses and reintegrates the human being into their earthly roots. Currently, several national and foreign research centers are dedicated to studying the substances present in medicinal plants. Science is beginning to surrender to the power of nature. Nature is present with us in every bit of ground with earth, light, air and water.

Types of Preparation

You can grow your own medicinal plants at home or in small spaces. The important thing is the healing energy you mentalize. Here are some important tips for collecting and preparing medicinal herbs: the plants should be harvested when wet and preferably on a full moon at dawn, wet with dew; dry the plants in the shade; then store them in a dry place separated by species; do not use them if mold or dampness appears.

Once you have obtained the herbs, keep them stored in glass or ceramic containers, away from dust, moisture and heat. If you buy them from somewhere, be aware of the quality and purity of the herbs, as well as whether they have been grown away from pesticides.

The best known ways of using medicinal plants are:

Tea: Traditional **tea:** the herb is poured into boiling water and left to boil for about 1/2 minute in a covered container. Leave it covered for a few minutes.

Infusion: boiling water is poured over the plants and the container is covered for 10 to 15 minutes. Ideal for flowers and leaves.

Decoction: the plant is boiled for a while in a covered container. Then leave it covered for a few minutes. This form is more suitable for roots, bark and seeds, but these should be cut into small pieces or crushed before use.

Maceration: the plant is soaked in cold water for up to 24 hours, depending on its quality. In this case, the vitamins and minerals are not altered by boiling.

The doses of herbs to be used vary greatly, but on average you can use 4 tablespoons of dried leaves per liter of water and 8 tablespoons of fresh leaves per liter of water. For roots and bark, it depends on the quality of the herb.

Tea should be taken pure or sweetened with pure honey, away from meals and several times a day.

Try swapping the coffee and chocolate for a cup of lemon balm, fennel, chamomile or mint, you'll feel much better!

Juices

They can be obtained by squeezing the leaves of the herbs through a thin cotton cloth, blending them in a blender or pounding them in a pestle. They are then strained and diluted with water and, if necessary, sweetened with honey. For adults, 5 drops per tablespoon of water is recommended.

Salads

Herbs can also be eaten raw in the form of salads or prepared with food as seasonings. However, great care must be taken with the quality and cleanliness of the herbs.

Wash them well under running water and then soak them for a while in water, sea salt and vinegar.

Dandelion, ox tongue, cow tongue, plantain, mint, parsley and yarrow are among the many good herbs for salads.

Baths

Some plants can be added to the warm water in the bath and the bath should last about 20 minutes.

Poultices

Fresh herbs can be applied loosely directly to the skin or supported by gauze.

They can also be crushed into a paste, placed between two thin cloths or gauze and applied to the affected area.

They can be used to treat neuralgia, earaches, asthma, cramps, etc.

Compresses

Cloths are soaked in a strong concentrated decoction and applied to the affected area. Hot teas have a sedative effect on swelling, neuralgia, bruising, rheumatism, gout, etc.

Gargling and Inhalations

Gargle a few times a day with tea prepared by decoction. This treatment acts on the oral cavity and throat.

To make inhalations, prepare a strong herbal tea, remove it from the heat, place an inverted paper funnel over the container, cover your head with a cloth and breathe in the evaporated air. Inhalations are great for treating flu, sinusitis, colds, pneumonia, etc.

Washing

The teas can also be used for intestinal washes, in the case of digestive disorders, and vaginal washes, for example in the case of discharge.

Dyes

The plants are cold macerated in grain alcohol at 60° or 70°.

Ointments

Prepared by mixing herbs with a greasy substance such as Vaseline.

Capsules, ointments, lozenges and tablets

Prepared by special techniques including crushing, pressing, extraction and others.

Comments:

Never use tea for more than 24 hours after it has been prepared, as it will ferment; and don't use the same type of tea for more than 30 days in a row, as your body will respond less and less.

Avoid preparing herbs in metal utensils, as they can cause changes in the effect and flavor of the tea due to oxygenation. Prefer clay, earthenware or enamel containers.

22 MEDICINAL PLANTS, GENERAL INDICATIONS

A Brief Compendium of Brazilian Herbal Medicines:

Avocado tree - Persea gratissima

Pulp, leaves, seeds and bark

Fruit pulp: antirachitic and aphrodisiac

Leaf infusion: diuretic, digestive, kidney and bladder, headaches, fever, bronchitis and tuberculosis.

Seeds: in poultice: abscesses; grated in alcohol: rheumatism.

Bark : vermifuge

Pineapple - Ananas sativus

Pulp and rind

Juice, tea and bark: diuretic, vermifuge, cough reliever and expectorant.

Pulp : digestive; external application: canker sores

Pumpkin - Cucurbita pepo

Pulp and seeds dried and toasted with salt.

Decoction of the pulp: diarrhea and gas.

Pulp juice : constipation.

Leaf poultice: burns, inflammations and earaches.

Fresh raw leaves, sautéed or powdered: anemia and avitaminosis.

Seeds: vermifuge.

Flowers : otitis.

Watercress - Nasturtium officinale

Leaves and flowers

Raw salads: exciting, fights scurvy, anemia, digestive and diuretic.

Against fever and toothache.

Infusion : bronchitis, depurative, diuretic, fever, jaundice.

Juice : fights smoke.

Celery - Aipum graveolens

Stem, leaves and root

Decoction of leaves and roots: diuretic, purifying and carminative. Arthritis, rheumatism, gallstones.

Seed infusion : gas, poor digestion

Artichoke - Cynara scolymus

Leaves and root.

Decoction and capsules : biliary calculi and liver disorders, diuretic, combats anemia, rickets, hemorrhoids, varicose veins and rheumatism, aid in weight loss regimes.

Garden Rosemary - Rosmarinus officinalis

Leaves and flowers - aromatic

Compresses: abscesses; rosemary + lavender compress: protects breasts during breastfeeding.

Rosemary smoke (steam) : coughs, bronchitis, asthma and flu.

Oil: hair loss.

Rosemary wine: diuretic, dropsy, physical and intellectual exhaustion.

Decoction and tincture : digestive, gas, fever, tiredness.

Baths : rheumatism.

Ointment : scabies, rheumatism.

Lettuce - Lactuca sativa

Fresh leaves

Poultice : bruises and swelling.

Decoctions : insomnia, calming and intestinal.

Lavender - Ocimum basilicum - Basil

Fresh or dried leaves

Infusion: bad mood, weakness, cramps and vomiting.

Leaves inside beans: intestinal gas.

Decoction : mouth and throat.

Lavender - Lavandula officinalis - Lavender

Dried leaves

Infusion : conjunctivitis.

Dried flowers

Infusion : asthma, bronchitis, pharyngitis, laryngitis, whooping cough, rheumatism, nervousness, insomnia, neuralgia, digestive, burns, migraine.

Massage oil: tiredness, bruises, stomachaches, vertigo, hemicrania.

Garlic - Allium sativum - Leek, common garlic and hortense garlic.

Bulb and stem

Ointment : corns

Oil and infusion : insomnia, hypertension, tuberculosis, colds, coughs, bronchitis, infectious wounds, lowers bad cholesterol.

Poultice : rheumatism

Decoction : worms

Note: Too much can cause stomach and headaches. Contraindicated for nursing mothers and people with low blood pressure.

Plum tree - Pronus domestica

Fresh leaves and ripe fruit

Plum liqueur : digestive

Fruit pulp : laxative and digestive

Infusion of leaves and dried fruit : cold, cough, hoarseness

Leaf poultice : vermifuge

Mulberry - Morus alba, Morus nigra

Fruit, leaves, bark and root

Gargle with infusion or juice of the fruit: canker sores, tonsillitis and toothache

Decoction of bark and roots : toothache, stomach, intestines, vermifuge

Leaf infusion : diuretic, hypertension

Syrup : cough, throat

Leaf poultice : eczema, skin rashes

Bath: invigorating.

Angelica - Angelica officinalis

Root, leaves, flowers and seeds

Infusion : digestive, diuretic, purifying, hysteria

Decoction : diarrhea

Beware: the leaves of the angelica are very similar to those of the poisonous hemlock.

Arnica - Arnica montana - Tabacode Savóia

Roots and flowers

Ointment: acne, boils

Infusion of flowers: stomach tonic

Tincture: bruises, falls, sprains, hematomas, rheumatic muscle pain.

Warning: Arnica is a poisonous plant, so oral administration of arnica-based medicines should be done under medical prescription.

Mastic

Bark and Leaves

Decoction: throat, wounds, tumors, inflammations in general. Bath: scabies and hemorrhoids.

Rice - Oryza sativa

Decoction for washing : hemorrhoids

Decoction : colitis, enteritis, intestinal infection

Rue - Ruta graveolens - Ruta sativa - Stinking rue, household and garden.

Fresh leaves

Leaf poultice : abscesses and otitis

Infusion of the leaves: gas, neuralgia, worms (in oil), migraine, lice, scabies, fleas.

Decoction of leaves for washing: eye inflammation

Note: Do not use during pregnancy.

Artemisia - Artemisia vulgaris

Leaves, flowers and roots

Powder : infantile convulsions, epilepsy

Infusion of leaves and flowers : painful menstruation, dysmenorrhea, fever, gout, rheumatism, worms

Leaves : "moxa" used in acupuncture treatment

Juice : women's diseases

Note: Do not use when pregnant or breastfeeding.

Assa-Peixe - Vernonia sp.

Leaves, flowers and fruit

Infusion : flu, bronchitis, asthma, coughs

Avenca - Adiantum capillus veneris - Venus's Hair; Common Avenca and Canada Avens

Leaves

Decoction and infusion: flu, cough, hoarseness, bronchitis, regulates menstruation.

External use: dandruff and hair loss In alcohol: warts.

Aloe vera

Internal use : stomachic and laxative

Juice - external use : antidandruff, antifungal, antibacterial, healing, repellent, glaucoma Suppository : hemorrhoid

Purslane - Portulaca oleracea

Leaves and seeds

Infusion of leaves : diuretic, eye inflammation

Salads and seeds : dewormer

External use : wounds

Chilean Bilberry - Peumus boldus

Leaves

Decoction : gallstones, stomach and liver disorders

Tea : tranquilizer, insomnia

Corn Hair - Corn Beard

Corn hair

Tea : diuretic, kidney stones, urinary infections, uric acid, albuminuria

Calendula officinalis - Calendula officinalis - Mal-me-quer - Verrucària

Flowers and leaves

Infusion : flu, scurvy, jaundice, eye inflammation, arthritis

External use : skin inflammations

Soaps : burns

Leaves : corns and warts

Cambarà - Lantana camarà- camarà

Flowers and leaves

Tea : coughs, colds, flu, bronchitis, asthma, whooping cough

Common chamomile - Matricaria chamomilla

Flowers

Infusion : fever, insomnia, neuralgia, colic, gas, indigestion, dyspepsia, lack of appetite, intestinal infections

Compresses and rinses : conjunctivitis, eye inflammation and tired eyes

Roman Chamomile - Anthemis nobilis

Same properties as regular chamomile, but stronger.

Cana-do-Brejo - Costus sp.

Cystitis, kidney infection, high blood pressure, circulation and enemas.

Lemongrass - Cymbopogon citratus Stapf

Leaves

Infusion: anxiety, hysteria, calming, gas, poor digestion. Infusion with honey and inhalation: bronchitis.

Carqueja - Baccharis trimera

Leaves

Infusion and capsules : organic weakness, liver, indigestion, diarrhea, lack of appetite, diabetes, rheumatism, gout, weight loss diets.

Sacred Mask - Rhammus purshiana

Bark

Decoction and capsules : liver, stomach, intestines, laxative, hemorrhoids.

Leather Hat - Echinodorus grandiflorus Mitch

Leaves

Decoction : rheumatism, urinary infections, pain, arthritis, atherosclerosis, diuretic, syphilis, depurative, gout External use and tea : dermatitis

Black tea - Thea sinensis - Indian tea - Chinese tea - Pekoe tea

Leaves

Infusion : stomatitis, poor digestion, cold, excitant, diuretic, analgesic, sudorific, nervous stimulant.

Onion - Allium cepa

Bulbs

Wine infusion: calluses, diuretic

Tincture : diuretic

Ointment : hemorrhoids, chilblains

Decoction : intestinal infections, constipation

Bulb : nosebleed, bee sting

Infusion : cold, cough, worms

Carrot - Daucus carota

Roots and seeds

Poultice : burns

Decoction : hoarseness, coughing

Confrey - Symphytum officinalis

Leaves, root

Tea : infections, bleeding, ulcers, leukemia, cuts and wounds Poultice : bone fractures, varicose veins, healing, ulcers, wounds, burns, anti-inflammatory, fractures

Copaiba

Resin - oil

Oil : syphilis, bronchitis, cough, dermatitis, urticaria, healing, ulcer, wounds, antiseptic, leucorrhea, urinary infections

Cloves - Eugenia Caryophyllata

Flowers

Tea and powder : excitant, toothache, digestive, aphrodisiac, purifying Wine infusion : bronchitis, flu, cough, colds

Dandelion - Taraxacum officinale

Flowers, leaves and roots

Salad : blood purifying, liver

Decoction and infusion : depurative, dropsy, liver disorders, acidosis, jaundice, diabetes

Leaf juice: kidney and liver stones. External use: vitiligo.

Whaling Grass - Cordia verbenacea - Catinga de Mulata

Leaves

Infusion, tincture and ointment: anti-inflammatory, back pain, rheumatism, cleansing and wound healing.

Lemongrass - Lippia sp.

Flowers and leaves

Infusion and tincture : ulcers, digestive, soothing, anti-inflammatory, respiratory tract, gas, jaundice, cardiac tonic.

Compresses : wounds

Bath : soothing

Fennel - Pimpinella anisum -Funcho - Aniseed

Seeds

Infusion: intestines, gas, colic, obesity, cramps, rheumatism, diabetes, eyes, memory, purifying, stimulates milk secretion. Olive oil - external use: lice

Monkey grass - Leonurus sibiricus L.

Leaves

Infusion: Heartburn, intestinal infection, powerful antibiotic, worms, diabetes.

Yerba Mate - Ilex paraguayensis / brasiliensis

Leaves

Infusion : exciting, invigorating, activates circulation, diuretic, digestive, laxative, dyspepsia, stomach and liver disorders

Bird's-foot trefoil - Struthanthus concinnus Mart.

Leaves and Flowers

Infusion: diabetes, hemorrhages, wound cleansing, ulcers, uterine diseases, pneumonia, asthma, high blood pressure.

Erva-de-Santa-Maria - Chenopodium ambrosioides- Vomiqueira - Ant grass

Leaves and seeds

Infusion and tincture : bronchitis, cough, diuretic, soothing, tuberculosis Juice : vermifuge

Note: Do not use during pregnancy. In large quantities it is poisonous.

Erva-de-Sâo-Joâo - Ageratum conysoides L. - Catinga de Bode

Leaves

Infusion : diarrhea, dysentery, colic and gas, rheumatism and depression.

Note: After using the infusion, do not expose yourself to the sun (wear a cap and glasses), as this can cause cataracts.

Espinheira Santa - Maytenus hicifolia- Lifeguard - Thorn of God

Leaves

Infusion and capsules : analgesic, disinfectant, healing, pain, gastritis, ulcer, laxative, diuretic Juice : wounds, acne, eczema

Note: Do not use during breastfeeding.

Eucalyptus - Eucalyptus globulus

Leaves

Inhalation - oil : asthma, bronchitis, healing, disinfectant

Leaf infusion : bronchitis, fever, stomatitis, pharyngitis, flu, cold, cough, sedative, disinfectant, sudorific, whooping cough, tuberculosis.

Massage oil diluted in almond or grape seed oil: rheumatic pain.

Ginger - Zingiber officinalis

Root and bark

Infusion, mashed root and crystals: excitant, dyspepsia, gas, diarrhea, flu, cough, bronchitis, cold, asthma, cholera, gout, infections, bad breath, tartar, gum inflammation, lowers cholesterol, stimulates immunity, aphrodisiac. Compress: bursitis.

Ginseng - Panax quinquefolium

Root

Infusion and mashed root: invigorating, colds, coughs, stomatitis, constipation, urinary and lung inflammations, nervous disorders, fatigue, gastric ulcers

Sunflower - Helianthus annus

Toasted leaves and seeds

Tincture of the leaves : fever, malaria, cold, stomatitis, hematuria

Seed infusion : nervous excitement

External use tincture : sores, contusions, wounds

Guava tree - Psidium guajava

Leaves

Poultice: varicose veins.

Juice: stomatitis.

Seat bath: vaginal discharge.

Sprouts

Infusion: diarrhea and dysentery.

Guaco - Mikania glomerata Spreng - Catinga vine

Leaves

Infusion and Tincture: rheumatism, arthritis, syphilis, gout

Decoction: respiratory and throat diseases.

Syrup: cough, flu.

Poultice: snakebite and poisonous insects.

Guaranà - Paullinia cupana

Seeds reduced to powder

Powder, refreshment, juice, capsule : invigorating, stimulating, infections, diarrhea, constipation, gas, disinfectant, arteriosclerosis, depression, hemorrhage, heart toning External use : wound healing

Note: children, pregnant or breastfeeding women, cardiac patients and hypertensive patients should avoid it.

Guinea - Petiveria alliacea

Leaves

Infusion: antispasmodic, abortifacient, diuretic, venereal diseases, vermifuge, rheumatism, spiritual protector.

Tincture and external bath: rheumatism.

Note: Contraindicated in pregnancy.

Witch hazel - Hamamelis virginiana

Bark and leaves

Witch hazel water: disinfectant

Decoction : diarrhea

Ointment and tincture : hemorrhoids, dysentery, gonorrhea, leucorrhea, tumors, external inflammations, plagues, eye inflammation, insect bites, varicose veins, excessive menstruation, pulmonary hemorrhage

Hyssop - Hyssopus officinalis

Dried flowers and leaves

Oil and infusion : asthma, bronchitis, inflammation of the mouth and throat, purifying, digestive

Oil and external use of infusion : sores and ulcers, skin rashes Compress : contusions

Mint - Monarda punctata

The whole plant

Infusion and salad : amenorrhea, nausea, vomiting, gas, analgesic, stimulant, diuretic

Peppermint - Mentha piperita

The whole plant

Oil and infusion : heart, poor digestion, insomnia, hepatic and abdominal colic, headaches, vermifuge, vomiting, cold, aphrodisiac

External use : rheumatism

Inhalation : asthma, cough, cold

Ointment : breastfeeding: prevents milk secretion

Leaf poultice : skin

Insulin - Cyssus sycioides - Climbing indigo, cipó-pucà

Leaves

Infusion: diabetes, rheumatism, abscesses, epilepsy, stroke, improves blood circulation.

Jurubeba - Solanum paliculatum

Leaves: healing.

Roots: Diabetes.

Fruits, leaves and roots: abscesses, uterine tumors.

Note: the fruit and roots can be toxic in large quantities.

Orange tree - Citrus aurantium

Bark, leaves, flowers and juice

Oil and flower infusion : stomatitis, insomnia, fever, calming.

Juice: digestive, ulcers, arthritis, constipation.

Lemon - Citrus limonum

Juice and rind of the fruit, leaves

Juice : gout, rheumatism, arteriosclerosis, hypertension, arthritis, blood purification, fever, wounds (external)

Gargle : mouth and throat inflammations

Infusion : poor digestion, gas, diarrhea, insomnia, conjunctivitis

Decoction : malaria

Friction : neuralgia, rheumatism

Wormwood - Artemisia absinthium - Absinthe - Worm weed

Dried leaves and flowers

Tincture of flowers and leaves : tonic, biliary and hepatic disorders, flatulence, poor digestion, soothing, rheumatism, gout, fever. Infusion of flowers : vermifuge

Macela - Achyrocline satureioides - Marcela

Flowers

Infusion: colic, diarrhea, upset stomach, calming. Bath: skin blemishes.

Apple tree - Pirus malus

Trunk bark and fruit

Apple water : urinary inflammation, poor digestion, acidity, fever, cold, hoarseness, diarrhea, constipation, soothing.

Sitz bath : leucorrhea

Apple wine: poor digestion, acidity

Mallow - Malva sylvestris

Dried flowers and leaves

Infusion and decoction of leaves and flowers : urinary infection, constipation, intestinal infection, obesity, coughs

Infusion of flowers - mouthwash: inflammation of the mouth, gums and throat Poultice of leaves: arthritis, gout, abscesses, teeth, ulcers, wounds, insect bites.

Flower and leaf bath : nervousness

Castor bean - Ricinus communis

Castor oil and leaves

Oil : hair, chilblains, constipation, vermifuge

Bath with a decoction of the leaves :hemorrhoids

Leaf poultice: tumors

Marjoram - Origanum majorana

Dried flowers

Oil and infusion : antispasmodic, stomach dilation, insomnia, gas Inhalation infusion : colds

Melissa - Melissa officinalis

Flowers and leaves

Infusion and tincture : anxiety, hysteria, hemicrania, gas, poor digestion

Compresses : wounds

Bath : soothing

Milleaf - Achillea millefolium- Milefolia

The whole plant

Infusion of leaves and flowers : diarrhea, urinary incontinence, hemorrhage, miscarriage prevention, gas

Infusion of leaves and flowers for poultice: sores, wounds, cracks in the breasts, hemorrhoids, ulcers, rheumatism, fever, varicose veins

Strawberry - Fragaria vesca

Leaves, roots and nuts

Root decoction : inflammation of the mouth and throat, intestines, diuretic, vermifuge

Compresses : sores, wounds, ulcers, small burns

Juice : toothache, fever, gout, stones

Note: Do not use in case of allergy or diabetes.

Pata-de-Vaca - Bauhinia sp.

Diabetes, kidney and urinary disorders.

Black Woodpecker - Bidens pilosa

Hepatitis and worms.

Pennyroyal - Mentha sp. - Erva de Sao Lourenço

Leaves

Infusion : coughs, **hoarseness**, stomach ailments, gas, bronchitis, asthma.

Stone - Phyllanthus niruri

Leaves, root and stem

Infusion and capsules: kidney and urinary infections, back pain, anuria, albuminuria, dropsy, kidney and biliary stones, discharge, hepatitis B.

Note: contraindicated in pregnancy; excessive consumption can lead to intoxication.

Rome - Punica granatum

Root, bark, leaves, flowers, pulp and bark of romas

Bark infusion: gums, sore throat, diuretic

Crumb : colic, diarrhea, tapeworm

Juice: fever, hemorrhoids, throat and angina.

White Garden Rose - Rosa canina, centifolia and gallica

Flower

Infusion : stomatitis, mouth and throat inflammation (gargling), poor digestion, diarrhea, constipation, bad breath, worms

Infusion for compresses : eyes

Rose vinegar for Washes : urticaria, bee stings, burns Washes : leucorrhea

Baths : energizing

Elderberry - Sambucus nigra

Root and flowers

Leaf poultice : abscesses, hemorrhoids

Infusion of leaves: diabetes

Infusion of flowers : breastfeeding: increases lacteal secretion, bronchitis, flu, eyes (washes), sudoriferous, measles, chicken pox, variola, scarlet fever. Decoction of bark and flowers: gout, uric acid, depurative, diuretic, dropsy, obesity, colds, kidneys, constipation.

Sage - Salvia officinalis

Leaves and flowers

Smoking : asthma

Decoction : stomatitis, mouth inflammations, whooping cough, heart, gums, cold sweats, coughs

Infusion : nervous exhaustion, poor digestion, kidney and liver stones, sore throat (gargle) Baths : tiredness

Stevia - Stevia rebaudiena

Leaves

Infusion : diabetes, diuretic, toning, rheumatism, hypertension, calming, insomnia, tension, digestive, inflammation, fever, obesity - sweetener

Plantain - Plantago lanceolata - Transage

Leaves and seeds

Poultice : sores , ulcers

Infusion and decoction: purifying, stomatitis, restorative, colds, ulcers of the throat and tongue, tonsillitis, fever, diarrhea, bronchitis.

Infusion for rinses : conjunctivitis, eye inflammations

Gargling : inflammation of the mouth, gums, throat

Nettle - Urtica dioica

Leaves, stems and seeds

Infusion : arthritis, dandruff (external use), epistaxis, hemorrhoids, uterine bleeding Decoction : depurative, boils, gout, hair loss (external use), diarrhea, hemorrhage

Infusions for external use : urticaria, rashes, itching

Note: may be toxic. Consult therapist before use.

Urucum - Bixa orellana

Seeds

Infusion: heart, constipation, bleeding and stomach ailments, cough and bronchitis

Violet - Viola odorata - Viola alba

Roots, leaves, dried flowers

Infusion and decoction : coughs, bronchitis, measles, sore throats, vomiting Cataplasm : bruises

Juniper - Juniperus communis - Junipero

Wood and berries

Infusion, decoction and oil: asthma, bronchitis, acidity, poor digestion, dropsy, diuretic

Alcoholate: rheumatism

23 PLANT SPECIES RECOMMENDED FOR TREATING DIABETES

Summary:

Diabetes mellitus is a chronic disorder caused by high blood sugar levels. WHO projections show that approximately 150 million people in the world have diabetes, and this number will probably double by 2025. Several species have been tested for their effectiveness in treating diabetes, such as *Taraxacum officinale* (dandelion), *Cynara scolymus* (artichoke), *Arctium lappa* (burdock), *Baccharis trimera* (carqueja), among others. In this study it was possible to observe that the 10 most cited plants for this pathology were *Allium cepa* (onion), *Phyllanthus niruri* (stone-breaker), *Arctium lappa* (burdock), *Taraxacum officinale* (dandelion), *Syzygium jambolanum*, *Stevia rebaudiana*, *Salvia officinalis, Eucalyptus globulus*, Baccharis *trimera*, *Bauhinia* forficata. In terms of the number of species per family, the most representative was the

FABACEAE (14 species); followed by ASTERACEAE (12 species), as well as the LAMIACEAE families (6),

MYRTACEAE and ROSACEAE (5), RUTACEAE and APIACEAE (4), SOLANACEAE (3), JUGLANDACEAE, SIMAROUBACEAE, GERANEACEAE, ERICACEAE, BRASSICACEAE, LILIACEAE and EUPHORBIACEAE (2). The results should contribute to ethnopharmacological screening and direct research into the use of Brazilian plants for the treatment of diabetes.

INTRODUCTION

Diabetes mellitus is a chronic disorder related to the absorption of glucose from the blood by cells (CLARE-SALZLER et al., 2003). Diabetes can appear as an autoimmune disease (type I) or as a disorder where insufficient insulin absorption is the main physio-pathological factor (type II). Type I diabetes is known as juvenile type and type II as adult-onset (www.diabetes.org.br).

Diabetes can appear without any clinical manifestations, years before the clinical picture of diabetes appears (FONSECA et al., 2005). WHO projections show that approximately 150 million people in the world have diabetes, and this number will probably double by 2025. The demonstration that this incidence can be reduced by lifestyle changes is hopeful, especially for those who have close relatives with the disease and its vascular complications: loss of vision, kidney failure, heart attack, stroke, sexual impotence, among others (WHO, 2005).

Since time immemorial there have been reports of the use of medicinal plants by man.

Based on popular use, scientific research has been carried out to prove their therapeutic effects. In order to be used safely, herbal medicines must meet the basic requirements of efficacy, safety and quality. Therefore, the evaluation of products obtained from plant drugs should primarily consider the identification of the drug by the pharmacopoeia (SHULTZ et al., 2002).

Numerous species have been tested for their efficacy in the treatment of diabetes, such as

Taraxacum officinale (dandelion), Cynara scolymus (artichoke), Arctium lappa (burdock), Baccharis trimera (carqueja), among other species (FUENTES et al., 2004). Different studies indicate that garlic (Allium sativum L.) contributes to stabilizing blood sugar levels (BALUCHNEJADMOJARAD & ROGHANI, 2003). Many herbs are known to affect blood sugar levels, which can cause a significant variation in the need for insulin. In Traditional Chinese Medicine, ginseng has shown good results in regulating blood sugar levels and is generally used to treat diabetes (XIE et al., 2005). The aim of this study is to review the literature on plant species indicated for the treatment of diabetes, in order to contribute to ethnopharmacological screening and to direct research into the potential of Brazilian species for the treatment of this pathology.

Data collection:

For the bibliographic survey, references were consulted with popular information and scientific books on the use of phytotherapy for the treatment of diabetes. Four scientific books, 12 popular books, seven websites and 19 scientific papers were consulted. Based on this survey, a table was constructed in which data was recorded on the species in relation to family, scientific name, popular name(s), part used, number of citations, citations in which they were found.

Data analysis:

The twelve families and ten species most cited in the literature were identified, and these were considered in terms of their potential for scientific study and therapeutic use. Scientific articles were searched in different databases to check the activity and toxicity studies of the ten most cited plants for the treatment of diabetes.

MOST COMMONLY USED HERBAL REMEDIES

A total of 106 species from 53 botanical families were cited in the literature as being useful in the treatment of diabetes. Table 1 contains data on the species found in the bibliographic survey. The 10 most cited species in the literature were *Allium cepa* (onion), *Phyllanthus niruri* (stone-breaker), *Arctium lappa* (burdock), *Taraxacum officinale* (dandelion), *Syzygium jambolanum*, *Stevia rebaudiana*, *Salvia officinalis, Eucalyptus globulus*, Baccharis *trimera*, *Bauhinia* forficata.

Table 1 - Results of the survey of plant species indicated in the literature for the treatment of diabetes (Annex 1).

Table 2 contains the ten most cited plants for treating diabetes.

Table 2- List of the ten most cited plants for treating diabetes.

(Popular name/Scientific name/Family)	No. of citations
Burdock *Arctium lappa* L. / ASTERACEAE	05
Dandelion *Taraxacum officinale* Weber ex F.H. Wigg. / ASTERACEAE	05
Onion *Allium cepa* L. / LILIACEAE	05
Stone breaker *Phyllanthus niruri* L. / EUPHORBIACEAE	05
Jambolan Syzygium jambolanum L / MYRTACEAE	05
Stevia Stevia rebaudiana (Bertoni) Bertoni / ASTERACEAE	05
Sàlvia *Salvia officinalis* L / LAMIACEAE	06
Eucalyptus Eucalyptus globulus Labill / MYRTACEAE	07
Carqueja *Baccharis trimera* (Less.) DC. / ASTERACEAE	09
Bauhinia forficata Link / FABACEAE	11

In terms of the number of species per family, the most representative was FABACEAE, with 14 taxa; followed by ASTERACEAE, with 12 taxa; as well as the families LAMIACEAE with 6 taxa, MYRTACEAE and ROSACEAE with 5 taxa; RUTACEAE and APIACEAE with 4 tàxons; SOLANACEAE with 3 tàxons; JUGLANDACEAE, SIMAROUBACEAE, GERANEACEAE, ERICACEAE, BRASSICACEAE, LILIACEAE, EUPHORBIACEAE and with 2 tàxons.

CONCLUSION ON HERBAL MEDICINE FOR DIABETICS

Phytotherapy is a science that can be applied to various pathologies. Research has been carried out with the aim of proving the effect of plant species that are often used only on the basis of empirical data. *Diabetes mellitus,* being a chronic disease with continuous treatment, is an interesting target for the search for new treatment methods.

Several species of medicinal plants can be used for the treatment of diabetes, contributing to ethnopharmacological screening and research into the potential of Brazilian species for the treatment of this pathological condition. The most cited plants in this study are included in several citations in published articles which reinforce the possible use of these plants in the treatment of *diabetes mellitus.*

Cow's foot (*Bauhinia forficata)*, one of the most cited species in this review, has been used in folk medicine to treat diabetes for a long time. The decoction can be used in the treatment of diabetes because it improves the condition without causing detectable tissue toxicity. Using some appropriate markers for the experimental model in rats, the extract of the plant was administered daily for seven days at doses of 200 and 400mg/kg, in diabetic and non-diabetic rats.

In conclusion, the results showed that the plant, when administered, can reduce glucose, triglycerides and total cholesterol. These results suggest the efficacy of the clinical use of this plant in the treatment of diabetes mellitus (PEPATO et al., 2004). (2002) demonstrated a significant reduction in glucose in the urine and serum of rats treated with *B. forficata.*) The crude extract of *B. candicans* showed hypoglycemic activity with a reduction in urinary glucose excretion, suggesting an increase in peripheral glucose metabolism (FUENTES et al., 2004).

Carqueja has the second highest number of citations for the treatment of diabetes. The aqueous fraction of *Baccharis trimera* showed potential anti-diabetic activity with a reduction in blood glucose after 7 days of treatment when used on diabetic rats (OLIVEIURA et al., 2005). In one study, crude extracts of carqueja (*Baccharis trimera*) and Jambolâo (*Syzygium cumini*) were used on diabetic and non-diabetic mice and treated for seven days. In this study, only fractions from twice-daily *Baccharis trimera* extracts reduced blood glucose after seven days of treatment. The results suggest that *Baccharis trimera* has a potent anti-diabetic activity (OLIVEIURA et al., 2005). No scientific studies were found on the use of the *Syzygium jambolanum* species.

Eucalyptus (*Eucalyptus globulus*) was administered as a decoction to mice, and a reduction in the level of hyperglycemia was observed (SWANSTON et al., 1990). Experiments have demonstrated the anti-hyperglycemic activity of eucalyptus, which is associated with the stimulation of insulin secretion, representing an additional treatment for the treatment of diabetes and demonstrating potential for the discovery of new active compounds for the treatment of diabetes (GRAY & FLATT, 1998).

The extract of *salvia* leaves (*Salvia officinalis*) showed a hypoglycemic effect in diabetic rats or mice and the plant should be considered for future research for therapeutic use (EIDI et al., 2005; ALARCON-AGUILAR et al., 2002).

Dandelion (*Taraxacum officinale*) did not affect glucose homeostasis parameters in mice (insulin and basal glucose levels, insulin-induced hypoglycemia, pancreatic pancreatic concentration) (SWANSTON-FLATT et al., 1989).

Stevia (Stevia rebaudiana) can be extracted from stevioside (a diterpene glycoside) which, when administered together with soy, seems to be an effective treatment for hyperglycemia in rats. Further studies are needed to verify that the results obtained in diabetic animals can be obtained in humans (DYRSKOG et al., 2005). Stevioside was able to regulate insulin deficiency in rats (CHEN et al., 2005) and reduce blood glucose in patients with type 2 diabetes, indicating beneficial effects on glucose metabolism (GREGERSEN et al., 2004).

Burdock (*Arctium lappa)* had no scientific citations in the sources used for this survey.

Despite being popularly cited, the lack of scientific citations on the use of burdock may be linked to the absence of a specific action in relation to *diabetes mellitus* and/or the presence of active substances in low concentrations to be tested.

Various studies have shown that *Allium cepa* (onion) has no hypoglycemic effect in the treatment of diabetic rats (JELODAR et al., 2005; EL-DEMERDASH et al., 2005).

Preparations with all parts of *Phyllanthus niruri* (stone-breaker) were administered for 10 days to patients with diabetes mellitus. The results indicated that this plant has a potential diuretic, hypotensive and hypoglycemic effect for humans (SRIVIDYA & PERWAL, 1995).

It is interesting to note that the Fabaceae family was the one with the highest number of species cited, this family being very important from a medicinal and economic point of view and the family to which *Bauhinia forficata* belongs, widely used in the treatment of diabetes and investigated *in in vitro* and *in vivo* trials.

The Asteraceae family was first described as Compositae by Dietrich Giseke. This family comprises 1528 genera, with approximately 22750 species found all over the planet. It is the largest botanical family among the angiosperms and is considered to be one of the largest sources of plant species of therapeutic interest, including *Cynara solymus* (artichoke) and *Baccharis trimera* (carqueja) (DI STASI & HIRUMA-LIMA, 2002).

The Lamiaceae family includes around 252 genera, in which 6700 species are distributed. In addition to its importance from a medicinal point of view, this family is also a source of species with great value as condiments, foodstuffs and in the perfume and cosmetics industry (DI STASI & HIRUMA-LIMA, 2002).

The results could help encourage research into new active compounds for the treatment of *diabetes mellitus*.

More investment is needed in scientific studies in this area in order to prove the effectiveness of these species as hypoglycemic agents.

24 AUTHOR'S CONSIDERATIONS:

This work was based on research in the databases of the USP School of Medicine and the USP School of Psychology, as well as a review of classes already taught in the Doctorate in Psychoanalysis. The aim was to produce material to help patients treated at university outpatient clinics and at my Physiotherapy and Psychoanalysis Clinic, which focuses on weight loss and eating disorders. Since I was 12 years old, I have been dedicating myself to therapies. Early on, I joined the Martial Arts where I learned Chiropractic, Phytotherapy, Naturalistic Therapies and Alternative Therapies, seeking mastery in physical, emotional and mental therapy. As my studies evolved, I was able to graduate as a Physiotherapist, where I specialized in Orthopedics and Rheumatology, Geriatrics and Gerontology, Phytotherapy and Clinical Nutrition, as well as Psychoanalytic Therapy, and I am also studying for a Master's Degree in Science at USP's Faculty of Medicine, as well as a Free Doctorate in Psychoanalysis. All this to reinforce everything I had already learned and started in my youth, to try to be faithful to my acquired knowledge, making it an efficient and practical treatment tool for those who come to me, uniting my vocation with my profession and lifestyle. This legacy I have shared with my students in the subjects I teach at universities in Sao Paulo, Brazil.

This phytotherapy work is the result of more than two decades of accompanying patients, whether in clinics using phytotherapics, in university classrooms teaching, on courses in various cities around the country, or on plantations advising on how to harvest. Always showing everyone that practice must be allied to research, and that the diversity of Brazilian herbal medicines requires a lot of study and constant updating. This work expresses the efforts to demonstrate this traditional, efficient therapy, which brings practical results for patients.

Antonio Rodriguez:

25 BIBLIOGRAPHICAL REFERENCES

ALONSO, J. **Tratado de Fitofârmacos e Nutracêuticos. Rosàrio/Argentina:Corpus Libros, 2004**

CARRICONDE, C. **Introduçâo ao Uso** de **Fitoteràpicos nas Patologias** de **APS**.Olinda: Centro Nordestino de Medicina Popular, 2002.

GULBERT, B; FERREIRA, J.L. P; ALVES, L. F; **Plant monographs**

Brazilian and acclimatized medicinal plants. Curitiba: Abifito, 2005.

LEITE, J. P. V. **Fitoterapia: bases cientificas e tecnoiógicas**. Sâo Paulo: Atheneu, 2009.

MATOS, F.J. A , LORENSI, H. **Plantas medicinais do Brasil: Nativas e Exóticas**. Nova Odessa, SP: Instituto Plantarum, 2002.

MILLS, S. KERRY, B. **Principles and Practice of Phytoteraphy: Modern Herbal Medicine.** London: Churchil Livingstone, 2000.

NEWALL, C.A, ANDERSON, L.A, PHILLIPSON, J.D. **Medicinal plants: a guide for health professionals. health professionals.** São Paulo: Premier, 2002. Translated by

Mirtes Frange de Oliveira Pinheiro.

PHILLIP, R.B. **Herbal-Drug interaction and adverse effects: an evidence based quick reference guide**. London: Medical Publish, 2004.

SILVA, R. C. **Plantas Medicinais na Saùde Bucai**. Vitória: Rozeli Coelho Silva, 2002.

SCHULZ, V., HANSEL, R.; TYLER, V. E. **Rational Phytotherapy: a guide to phytotherapy for the health sciences.** Manole. São Paulo, 2002. Translated by Glenda M. de Sousa. MARTINS ER. Medicinal Plants. Viçosa: Editora UFV; 2000.

MATOS FJA. Farmàcias vivas: a system for using medicinal plants designed for small communities. Fortaleza: Editora UFC, 3. ed.; 1998.

Poetic Minute. Medicinal Plants. http:// www.minuto.poetico.nom.br (accessed on 07/Sep/2005).

OLIVEIURA AC, ENDRINGER DC, AMORIM LA, BRANDAO MD, COELHO MM. Effect of the extracts and fractions of *Baccharis trimera* and *Syzygium cumini* on glycaemia of diabetic and non-diabetic mice. *J Ethnopharmacol* . v.28, (epub ahead of print), 2005.

PEPATO MT, KELLER EH, BAVIERA AM, KETTELHUT IC, VENDRAMINI RC, BRUNETTI IL. Anti-diabetic

activity of *Bauhinia forficata* decoction in stretozotocin-diabetic rats. *J Ethnopharmacol.* v.81, n.2, p.191-7, 2002.

PEPATO MT, BAVIERA AM, VENDRAMINI RC, BRUNETTI IL. Evaluation of toxicity after one-months treatment with *Bauhinia forficata* decoction in stretozotocin-induced diabetic rats. *BMC Complementary and Alternative Medicine*. v.4, p.1-7, 2004.

RioNet. Canto Verde. http://www.rionet.com.br/~cantoverde/p.html (accessed on 07/Sep/2005).

RIQUEIRO MP. Plantas que Curam: Manual Ilustrativo de Plantas Medicinais. Publisher: Paulus, 6ª ed; 1992.

SCHULTZ, V, HANSEL R, TYLER VE. Rational phytotherapy: a guide to phytotherapy for the health sciences. Sao Paulo: Editora Manole, 2002; p.386.

SPETHMANN CN. Alternative Medicine from A to Z. Editora Natureza, 7ª edition; September 2004.

SRIVIDYA N, PERIWAL S. Diuretic, hypotensive and hypoglycaemic effect of *Phyllanthus amarus. Indian J Exp Biol* . v.33, n.11, p.861-4, 1995.

SWANSTON-FLATT SK, DAY C, FLATT PR, GOULD BJ, BAILEY CJ.

Glycaemic effects of traditional european plant treatments for diabetes, studies in normal and streptozocin diabetic mice. *Diabetes Res.* v.10, n.2, p.69-73, 1989.

SWANSTON-FLATT SK, DAY C, BAILEY CJ, FLATT PR. Traditional plant treatments for diabetes. Studies in normal and streptozotocin diabetic mice.

Diabetologia. v.33, n.8, p.462-4, 1990.

USP. Medicinal, Aromatic and Condiment Plants. http://www.ci-66.ciagri.usp.br/pm/index.asp(accessed 07/Sep/2005).

WILLIANS, T. Fitoterapia: Guia Pràtica. Publisher: Callis Ltda; 1998.

World Health Organization. Diabetes: the cost of diabetes.

http://www.who.int/mediacentre/factsheets/fs138/en/ (accessed on 07/Sep/2005).

XIE JT, WANG CZ, WANG AB, WU J, BASILA D, YUAN CS. Antihyperglycemic effects of total ginsenosides from leaves and stem of Panax ginseng. *Acta Pharmacol Sin.* v.26, n.9, p.1104-10, 2005.

YWATA C, ANTÔNIO J, CORDEIRO R. Medicina Natural - A Cura está na Natureza. Editora Três.

ALARCON-AGUILAR FJ, ROMAN-RAMOS R, FLORES-SAENZ JL, AGUIRRE-GARCIA F. Investigation on the hypoglycaemic effects of extracts of four mexican medicinal plants in normal and alloxan-diabetic mice. *Phytother Res.* v.16, n.4, p.383-6,2002.

Aquimia Vilabol. Medicinal plants. http://www.aquimia.vilabol.uol.com.Br/plantasmedicinais/page5.html (captured on September 7, 2005).

BALBACH A. *Fruits in Domestic Medicine*. Itaquaquecetuba: Editora Missionària, 1992 a.

BALBACH A. *Vegetables in Domestic Medicine*. Itaquaquecetuba: Editora Missionària, 1992 b.

BALBACH A. The Plants Heal. Sao Paulo: Vida Plena, 1993.

BALUCHNEJADMOJARAD T, ROGHANI M. Edothelium-dependent and independent effect of aqueous extract of garli on vascular reactivity on diabetic rats. *Fitoterapia*. v.74. n.7-8, p. 630-7, 2003.

BOARIM DS. Practical Manual of Natural Treatments. Vida Plena Editions, 1ª ed; 1998.

BRANDÂO MGL. Belo Horizonte Medicinal and Aromatic Plants Circuit.

CELiLIO, A. B. et al./Revista Eletrônica de Farmàcia Vol 5(3),23-28,2008.

CHEN TH, CHEN SC, CHAN P, CHU YL, YANG HY, CHENG JT. Mechanism of the hypoglycemic effects of stevioside, a glycoside of *Stevia rebaudiana*. *Planta* Med. v.71. n.2, p.108-13, 2005.

CLARE-SALZLER MJ, CRAWFORD JM, KUMAR V. The Pancreas. In: Kumar V, Cotran RS, Robbins SL, eds. Basic Pathology 7ª ed. Philadelphia: Saunders Publishing, 2003. p.635-655.

CORRÊA AD, BATISTA RS, QUINTAS LEM. Plantas medicinais: do cultivo à terapêutica. Petrópolis: Editora Vozes, 4.ed; 2001.

DI STASI LC, HIRUMA-LIMA CA. *Plantas medicinais na Amazônia e na Mata Atlântica*, 2nd ed. Sao Paulo: Editora Unesp, 2002. 605p.

DYRSKOG SE, JEPPESEN PB, COLOMBO M, ABUDULA R, HERMANSEN K. Preventive effects of a soy-based diet supplemented with stevioside onthe development of the metabolic syndrome and type 2 diabetes in Zucker diabetic fatty rats. *Metabolism*. v.54, n.9, p.1181-8, 2005.

Educa Terra. Medicinal Plants.

http://www.educaterraterra.com.br/almanaque/ciencia/plantas_medicinaisZ (accessed on 07/Sep/2005).

EIDI M, EIDI A, ZAMANIZADEH H. Effect of *Salvi alis* L. Leaves on serum glucose and insulin in healthy and streptozotocin-induced diabetis rats. *J Ethnopharmacol*. v.100, n.3, p.310-3, 2005.

EL-DEMERDASH FM, YOUSEF MI, EL-NAGA NI. Biochemical study on the hypoglycemic effects of onion and garlic in alloxan-induced diabetic rats. *Food Chem Toxicol*. v.43, n.1, p.57-63, 2005.

FETROW CW, AVILAJR. Handbook of alternative medicine for the professional. Rio de Janeiro: Editora Guanabara Kooga; 2000.

FONSECA CT, AMARAL DM, RIBEIRO, MG, BESERRA IC, GUIMARAES MM. Insulin resistance in adolescents with Down syndrome: a cross-sectional study. *BMC Endocr Disord*. v.17, p. 5-6, 2005.

FRANCOIJ, FONTANA UL. Herbs and Plants: The Medicine of the Simple. Erexim, R.S.: Editora Edebra, 7ª ed; 2002.

FUENTES O, ARANCIBIA-AVILA P, ALARCON J. Hypoglycemic activity of Bauhinia candicans in diabetic induced rabbits. *Fitoterapia*. v.75, n.6, p.527-32, 2004.

FUENTES O, ARANCIBA-AVILA P, ALARCON J. Hypoglycemic activity of *Bauhinia candicans* in diabetic induced rabbits. *Fitoterapia*. v. 75, n.6, p.527-32, 2004.

GRAY AM, FLATT PR. Antihyperglycemic actions of *Eucalyptus globulus* (Eucalyptus) are associated with pancreatic and extra-pancreatic effects in mice. *Bioch Mol Roles of Nutrients*. p.2319-2323, 1998.

GREGERSEN S, JEPPESEN PB, HOLST JJ, HERMANSEN K. Antihyperglycemic effects of stevioside in type 2 diabetic subjects. *Metabolism*. v.53, n.1, p.73-6, 2004.

JELODAR GA, MALEKI M, MOTADAYEN MH, SIRUS S. Effect of fenugreek, onion and garlic on boold glucose and histopathology of pancreas of alloxan- induced diabetic rats. *Indian J Med Sci*; v.59, n.2, p.64-9, 2005.

Language of Flowers. Organic products. http://linguagemdasflores.blogs.sapo.pt/arquivo/2004_04.html (accessed on 07/Sep/2005).

MARTINS ER. Medicinal Plants. Viçosa: Editora UFV; 2000.

MATOS FJA. Farmàcias vivas: a system for using medicinal plants designed for small communities. Fortaleza: Editora UFC, 3. ed.; 1998.

Poetic Minute. Medicinal Plants. http:// www.minuto.poetico.nom.br (accessed on 07/Sep/2005).

OLIVEIURA AC, ENDRINGER DC, AMORIM LA, BRANDAO MD, COELHO MM. Effect of the extracts and fractions of *Baccharis trimera* and *Syzygium cumini* on glycaemia of diabetic and non-diabetic mice. *J Ethnopharmacol* . v.28, (epub ahead of print), 2005.

PEPATO MT, KELLER EH, BAVIERA AM, KETTELHUT IC, VENDRAMINI RC, BRUNETTI IL. Anti-diabetic activity of *Bauhinia forficata* decoction in stretozotocin-diabetic rats. *J Ethnopharmacol.* v.81, n.2, p.191-7, 2002.

PEPATO MT, BAVIERA AM, VENDRAMINI RC, BRUNETTI IL. Evaluation of toxicity after one-months treatment with *Bauhinia forficata* decoction in stretozotocin-induced diabetic rats. *BMC Complementary and Alternative Medicine*. v.4, p.1-7, 2004.

RioNet. Canto Verde. http://www.rionet.com.br/~cantoverde/p.html (accessed on 07/Sep/2005).

RIQUEIRO MP. Plantas que Curam: Manual Ilustrativo de Plantas Medicinais. Publisher: Paulus, 6ª ed; 1992.

SCHULTZ, V, HANSEL R, TYLER VE. Rational phytotherapy: a guide to phytotherapy for the health sciences. São Paulo: Editora Manole, 2002; p.386.

SPETHMANN CN. Alternative Medicine from A to Z. Editora Natureza, 7ª edition; September 2004.

SRIVIDYA N, PERIWAL S. Diuretic, hypotensive and hypoglycaemic effect of *Phyllanthus amarus*. *Indian J Exp Biol* . v.33, n.11, p.861-4, 1995.

SWANSTON-FLATT SK, DAY C, FLATT PR, GOULD BJ, BAILEY CJ.

Glycaemic effects of traditional european plant treatments for diabetes, studies in normal and streptozocin diabetic mice. *Diabetes Res.* v.10, n.2, p.69-73, 1989.

SWANSTON-FLATT SK, DAY C, BAILEY CJ, FLATT PR. Traditional plant treatments for diabetes. Studies in normal and streptozotocin diabetic mice. *Diabetologia.* v.33, n.8, p.462-4, 1990.

USP. Medicinal, Aromatic and Condiment Plants. http://www.ci-66.ciagri.usp.br/pm/index.asp(accessed 07/Sep/2005).

WILLIANS, T. Fitoterapia: Guia Pràtico. Publisher: Callis Ltda; 1998. diabetes.

WorldHealthOrganization . Diabetes: in

thecostof

XIE JT, WANG CZ, WANG AB, WU J, BASILA D, YUAN CS. Antihyperglycemic effects of total ginsenosides from leaves and stem of Panax ginseng.

Acta Pharmacol Sin. v.26, n.9, p.1104-10, 2005.

YWATA C, ANTÔNIO J, CORDEIRO R. Medicina Natural - A Cura está na Natureza. Editora Três.

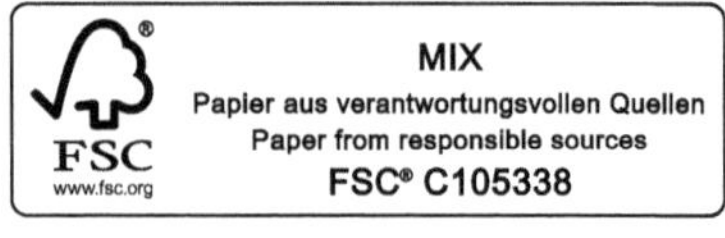

Printed by Books on Demand GmbH, Norderstedt / Germany